Bo Krasse   Caries Risk

Caries Risk
A Practical Guide for Assessment and Control

Bo Krasse, D.D.S., Odont. Dr.
Professor of Cariology
University of Göteborg
Göteborg, Sweden

Quintessence Publishing Co., Inc. 1985
Chicago, London, Berlin, Rio de Janeiro and Tokyo

Library of Congress Cataloging in Publication Data

Krasse, Bo.
  Caries risk.

  Translation of: Karies risk.
  Bibliography: p.
  Includes index.
  1. Dental caries—Diagnosis. 2. Dental caries—
Prevention. I. Title. [DNLM: 1. Dental Caries—
diagnosis. 2. Dental Caries—prevention & control.
3. Probability. WU 270 K89ka]
RK331.K7313 1985   617.6'7   84-26509
ISBN 0-86715-123-4

© 1985 by Quintessence Publishing Co., Inc., Chicago, Illinois.
All rights reserved.

This book or any part thereof must not be reproduced by any means or without the written permission of the publisher.

Composition: Compositors, Cedar Rapids, IA
Printing and binding: BookCrafters, Chelsea, MI
Printed in U.S.A.

Contents

Introduction		11
Chapter 1	**A Short Review of Pathogenesis**	15
Chapter 2	**Case History and Clinical Examination**	29
Chapter 3	**Dietary Analysis**	35
Chapter 4	**Salivary Examination**	41
Chapter 5	**Microbiological Examination**	45
Chapter 6	**Assessment of Findings**	49
Chapter 7	**Managing Dietary Problems**	53
Chapter 8	**Treating Poor Salivary Values**	59
Chapter 9	**Reducing Cariogenic Microorganisms**	63
Chapter 10	**Fluoride Prevention in Adults**	69
Chapter 11	**Principles of Treatment: Case Studies**	75
Chapter 12	**Identifying Risk Groups**	85
Chapter 13	**General Discussion**	91
Chapter 14	**Summary**	95
Further Reading		97
Index		102
Color Atlas		105

Foreword

Although incidence of coronal caries has been declining in most Western industrialized countries during the last two decades, some patients still experience extensive decay. Epidemiological surveys have shown that the decrease in decay has not been uniform and that about 20% of the population experience 60% of the caries increment. Identifying this high-risk group is not simply a theoretical problem in disease epidemiology but is of major importance from a clinical point of view, particularly in diagnosis and treatment planning.

The faculty in the Department of Cariology at the University of Göteborg have been using a combination of examinations to assess the caries risk of their patients. These examinations include past dental history, a medical history, history of fluoride exposure, personal history, and diet history. In addition, laboratory examinations are performed to determine salivary secretion rate and buffer capacity, as well as counts of *Streptococcus mutans* and lactobacilli. We in the dental profession are extremely fortunate that Professor Bo Krasse has made the effort to share with us his wealth of experience with these methods and his insights into their clinical relevance. It is high time that such information be extended from the research laboratories and the academic ivory towers to dental practitioners. Some of the tests described in this book are well within the capability of the private dental office, while other tests are best referred to a university, hospital, or clinical microbiological laboratory. Only by gathering all available information can we make an informed and intelligent judgment concerning treatment planning or assess the progress of preventive therapy. To do less would be a disservice to our patients.

Ernest Newbrun
Professor of Oral Biology
University of California at San Francisco

Preface

Microbial and salivary analyses are valuable adjuncts to the clinical and radiographic assessment of caries risk. They can also help monitor the effectiveness of caries preventive measures. This handbook describes and outlines simple methods for microbial and salivary analyses, as well as other methods of caries control. The knowledge summarized is the result of years of research and practice at the University of Göteborg, Sweden.

Most of the methods described have long been employed at dental schools all over the world. In general dental practice, however, they are rarely used at all. Since one explanation could be the unavailability of a simple handbook on the subject, I decided to write this book. It was published in Swedish in 1981, at the same time the Swedish Social Board announced its Dental Health Care Program for Adults. The board recommended that salivary and microbiological examinations be used whenever a high caries risk was suspected or extensive restorative treatment was planned. Swedish authorities now consider these examinations so important that patients are refunded 50% of their cost by the Government Insurance Office.

This English translation was spurred by a great international interest in the Swedish dental health system, a growing concern among dentists and laymen for prevention of caries, and by the enthusiastic response to the original Swedish version.

Caries Risk is not a textbook on cariology. It is intended primarily as a manual for dentists, dental students, and auxiliaries. I hope it will stimulate more widespread application of existing knowledge in the diagnosis, treatment, and prevention of caries.

Acknowledgments

I would like to thank my collaborators in research at the University of Göteborg: C. G. Emilson, Birgitta Köhler, Mona Svanberg, and Ingegerd Zickert.

This translated version was completed during a sabbatical year at the University of British Columbia. I would like to sincerely thank all who assisted me: Professor Barry C. McBride, Linda Skibo, Sally Wong, Dr. Nancy E. Schwarz, Dr. Lance M. Rucker, Dr. Ernest Newbrun, and Dr. William H. Bowen.

My special appreciation goes to Dr. George S. Beagrie, dean of the Faculty of Dentistry. He not only strongly supported and encouraged me in this venture, but also found the time in a busy schedule to transform my broken "Swenglish" into a readable language.

Introduction

The treatment of symptoms and the treatment of causes of disease should be separate. To control the development of or the recurrence of a disease, preventive measures must be taken.

Dental caries traditionally has been treated symptomatically. Carious lesions detected in teeth by routine examination or because of discomfort are treated. The carious material is removed, and the lost tooth substance is replaced by a filling or a crown. In the last few years, however, more and more interest has been focused on treatment of the cause.

Correct treatment of dental caries demands an adequate diagnosis. This means that there is a need to record not only the number of cavities, but also their location and appearance. Factors and conditions that might influence the disease activity, and the subsequent treatment and prevention of the disease, also have to be taken into account.

The diagnosis of dental caries—just as the diagnosis of any other disease—should be based on history, current state, and—if necessary—completing examinations. In this book, the main emphasis is put on the use of laboratory examinations as a supplement to history and current state. A thorough description of the dental caries state, however, is the basis for an adequate diagnosis. Commonly used terms are described here.

Caries prevalence or caries frequency

Caries prevalence or *caries frequency* gives the total number of teeth or tooth surfaces with caries in a population, regardless of whether they have been treated or not. The most common way to record this is by the DMFT or DMFS system (decayed, missing, and filled teeth; decayed, missing, and filled surfaces). When using the system, an extracted tooth or a tooth with a full crown represents four or five surfaces,

Introduction

depending on whether it is an anterior front tooth or a premolar or molar that is missing or has a crown.

In prevalence studies, the percentage of persons with caries in a population is often used, and sometimes the percentage of decayed teeth or tooth surfaces is given.

In order to determine whether the caries prevalence in one person is in agreement with the expected value, a comparison has to be made with data from studies on populations of the same age and of similar ethnic and socioeconomic background. In Table 1, the figures serve as a guideline for a rough estimate of the caries prevalence in an individual residing in a particular community.

Caries activity or caries incidence

Caries activity is—in broad terms—the speed with which the dentition is destroyed by caries. In mathematical terms, it represents the sum of new carious lesions and enlarged lesions per unit of time. If a large number of new lesions have developed within a short period of time, the caries activity is considered to be high.

However, even if no carious lesions are recorded at the clinical examination, the caries activity might still be high. It takes a certain period of time for the carious lesions to

Table 1 Caries prevalence (DMFT) in various age groups in different countries[*]

Age	Sweden	Canada
20	17	15
40	22	18
60	24	20

Age	U.S.A. (Baltimore)	Australia (Sydney)	Germany (Hanover)	Japan (Yamanashi)
35–44	16	19	15	11

[*]From A. Hugosson and G. Koch, 1979; D. E. Barmes, 1978; and a "Report on the Working Group on Preventive Services," Canada, 1980.

develop and reach a stage at which they can be registered clinically. Thus, strong caries-promoting factors may be present although no lesions are detected. For this reason, a new term has come into use: *actual caries risk.*

Actual caries risk

Actual caries risk describes to what extent a person at a particular time runs the risk of developing carious lesions. In most instances, the actual caries risk is generally considered "high" or "low." The evaluation is based on history, current state, and completing examinations.

Patient at risk

A *patient at risk* is a person with a high potential to contract a disease due to genetic or environmental conditions. A person or a group of persons at high dental caries risk will most likely be affected by caries attack. A person who has a large number of cavities is not necessarily at high dental caries risk. Such a person is already dentally ill and should be treated for the disease. This treatment must then be supported by preventive measures in order to avert the recurrence of the disease.

Preventive treatment

Preventive treatment is aimed at reducing the risk of illness or recurrence of the disease. For example, extraction of a tooth in order to reduce food retention and, with that, the caries risk is preventive treatment. On the other hand, oral hygiene instruction and prescription of fluoride rinsings for patients who do not have caries are *preventive measures* or called simply *prevention.*

Introduction

Diagnosis

Diagnosis (from Latin meaning "by knowledge") is the act of identifying a disease by its signs and symptoms.

The description of the state of the teeth not only should comprise a recording of the number of carious lesions and earlier dental treatment (i.e., the DMFT or DMFS of an individual), but also should include the location and appearance of the lesions present. For example, these questions should be answered: Are the lesions soft and light brownish, or hard and dark pigmented? On which surfaces of the teeth are the lesions situated? Do they occur on surfaces not earlier decayed (primary caries) or are they connected with earlier restorations (secondary caries)? Which type of lesions are dominant at the time of the examination should also be recorded.

In a new patient, it might be difficult to assess the caries activity, as the criteria for diagnosis of a lesion might vary among examiners. Furthermore, the date for the preceding examination might be uncertain. In patients who are recalled to the same dentist on a regular basis, these problems to a large extent are eliminated, because the dentist is familiar with their oral health status and should have records.

Finally, the diagnosis ought to include an evaluation of the actual caries risk.

Chapter 1

A Short Review of Pathogenesis

Dental caries is generally defined as a localized destruction of the teeth (the Latin word "caries" means decay).

The destruction of tissue in the enamel, 95% of which consists of the inorganic material hydroxyapatite, is caused mainly by organic acids, especially lactic acid. The acids are produced by microorganisms on the tooth surface which ferment carbohydrates, particularly sugars.

In the dentin, which contains about 20% collagenlike organic material, the demineralization is accompanied by a digestion of the organic structure.

Invasion of the enamel and underlying dentin by microorganisms can be more advanced than would be expected from the clinical examination. For example, underneath an initial carious lesion (chalky enamel) microorganisms can be found in the deeper parts of the enamel and sometimes also in the dentin. Destruction of the tooth mineral can be seen around these microorganisms.

The occlusal surface of the tooth is usually attacked first. There the decay starts in the fissures, where microorganisms often become entrapped as the tooth erupts. Microorganisms that colonize the smooth surface of the tooth must have specific properties in order not to be removed by the cleansing action of saliva or by chewing. Only a few of all the species found in the oral cavity have the ability to adhere to the teeth, and of these a limited group is cariogenic.

The initial carious lesion is characterized by a loss of translucence of the enamel which takes on a chalklike appearance. This stage is often called chalky enamel caries. The surface feels rough when probed. Probing, however, should be avoided. Parts of the crystal structure might be broken off and this impairs the possibilities for remineralization. Furthermore, cariogenic microorganisms which often occur in abundance in chalky enamel might attach to the tip of the dental explorer and be forced into a fissure that is probed afterwards. Another reason to not probe unnecessarily is that visual examination alone gives about the same information as a combined visual-tactile examination.

In the dentin, a rapidly progressing carious lesion is characterized by a soft, moist appearance; the color is light brown (see Figs. 10a and b in color atlas). A pigmented, dark brownish to black appearance (see Figs. 9a and b in color atlas) indicates a slow progression of the lesion. This type of caries is commonly termed arrested or chronic caries in contrast to acute caries.

When the salivary secretion rate is reduced, carious lesions often appear at the cementoenamel junction. In general, such carious lesions can be distinguished easily from erosions or idiopathic resorptions. These lesions, as a rule, have a hard base. On exposed root surfaces, carious lesions often expand in width first and do not show a distinct delineation. When preparing a cavity, it is often difficult to obtain a definite form of a box.

Table 2 Changes in caries prevalence among teenagers from different parts of the world[*]

Country	Age	DMFT	
Sweden	13	6.2 (1966)	3.4 (1978)
Canada	13	12.4 (1958)	6.99 (1980)
U.S.A.	12	13.1 (1958)	6.7 (1978)
Ethiopia	12	0.2 (1958)	1.5 (1975)
Japan	12	2.8 (1957)	5.9 (1975)
Italy	12	3.0 (1966)	6.9 (1977)

[*]From Mansson et al., 1979; British Columbia Children's Dental Survey, 1980; Glass, 1982; Barmes, 1980; and Infirri and Barmes, 1979.

A Short Review of Pathogenesis

Dental caries has been described as a serious sociomedical problem because the disease attacks almost 100% of the population. As with some other human diseases the pattern of dental caries has undergone changes with time. In the industrial countries the prevalence of caries in children and adolescents is showing a definite downward trend. By contrast, because of an increased access to dental care more teeth are being retained in the older age groups and, in these, more cases of dental caries in the roots of teeth are being recorded.

The dental caries picture in the developing countries is reported by epidemiologists to be the opposite with a dramatic increase in adolescents, which is mainly attributed to exposure to a Western-type diet.

Dental caries changes in various parts of the world are illustrated below and in Table 2. It should be noted that among military recruits in Sweden the number of DMFSs decreased to 21 in 1978 from 39 in 1958, whereas for teenagers in Sweden the decrease in DMFTs dropped to 3.4 in 1978 from 6.2 in 1966. On the other hand, in developing countries such as Ethiopia the DMFT rate has increased to 1.5 in 1975 from 0.2 in 1958.

Caries prevalence (DMFS) among military recruits in Sweden (Koch, 1982)

1958	1972	1981
39	29	21

Opinions differ as to the causes of caries reduction in the industrial countries. Some subscribe to an increased tooth resistance due to an increased use of fluorides, whereas others argue for reduced caries-promoting factors due to changes in dietary habits. It also seems possible that a widespread use of fluoride toothpaste may have led to changes of the oral microflora in such a way that cariogenic microorganisms of low virulence increased to the detriment of highly virulent strains and lessened the caries risk as a result.

A Short Review of Pathogenesis

Main factors

For caries to develop, the three main factors of host, microflora, and diet have to not only be present but also interacting (Fig. 1). This simple fact cannot be stressed strongly enough. The importance of observing the relationship between these three factors for the diagnosis, treatment, and prevention of caries will be emphasized continuously.

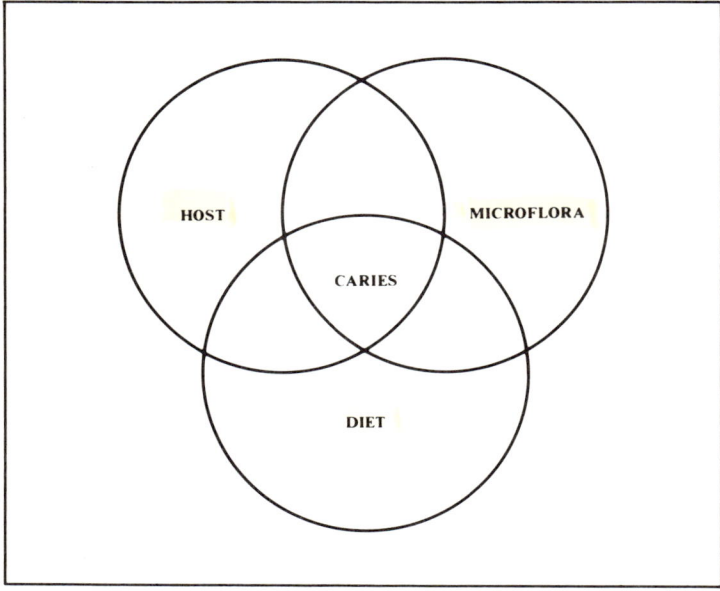

Fig. 1 The three main factors of host microflora and diet have to interact for dental caries to occur.

For evaluation of caries risk it is important that as many relevant facts as possible within each of the three circles of the diagram in Fig. 1 are recorded. Some of the facts can be measured objectively, whereas others have to be assessed. To a large extent, microbiological methods are used here, and in this short review, only essential information will be given as a background to such methodology.

Main Factors

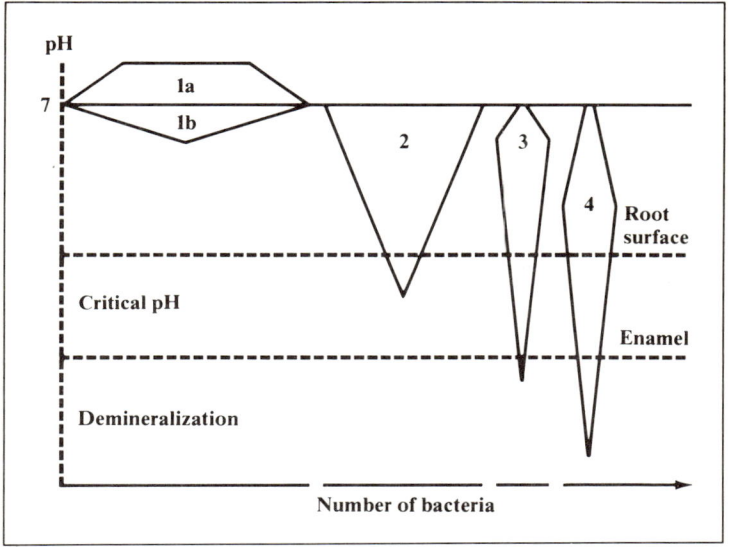

Fig. 2 It is the function of the microorganisms and not the total number of plaque bacteria that determines whether or not demineralization will occur.

Specific microorganisms

Some microorganisms are more important than others in the pathogenesis of dental caries, namely *Streptococcus mutans,* lactobacilli, and some *Actinomyces* species. *S. mutans* is generally associated with the initial development of caries, lactobacilli with the further development of the lesion, and *Actinomyces* with root surface caries.

Both lactobacilli and *S. mutans* have the capacity to grow and produce substantial amounts of acids at a low pH of around 5.0. This pH level can occur in dental plaque after fermentation of sugar to organic acids or by intake of acidic fruits and beverages. Low pH values favor the establishment of *S. mutans* on the tooth surface. The ability to grow and produce acid at a low pH is of ultimate importance in the role of a microorganism for the development of caries. Such has been demonstrated in a number of studies.

Figure 2 shows the acid production of different microorganisms in the plaque. Some of the bacteria might produce alkali (1a), others only slight amounts of acids (1b). Other microorganisms (2) comprise a large proportion of the total number of the plaque bacteria which, although they produce large amounts of acid, never cause the pH to reach the so-called critical level. The critical pH is the level at which the tooth substance is dissolved to a considerable degree; this level is believed to be between pH 5.3 and 5.7. Some microorganisms, such as *S. mutans* and lactobacilli (3 and 4), show optimal growth at a lower pH than other plaque bacteria and reach a final pH below the critical level.

It is evident from Fig. 2 that it is not the *number* of microorganisms but the functions of certain bacteria that determine whether demineralization will occur or not. Thus, in order to evaluate caries risk, the plaque index of a patient is of limited value. Instead, what has to be resolved is the extent to which a person is carrying caries-inducing microorganisms such as lactobacilli and *S. mutans*.

Streptococcus mutans

A considerable amount of research has been done on *S. mutans*. During the last decade, more than 700 original articles have been published that support the relationship between *S. mutans* and caries (van Houte, 1980; Newbrun, 1983). The most important are:

1. *S. mutans* induces dental caries in experimental animals such as hamsters, rats, and subhuman primates.
2. Correlation has been found between the presence of *S. mutans* in saliva and plaque material and the incidence of dental caries.
3. Infection of a tooth surface with *S. mutans* generally precedes the development of caries.
4. More surfaces are infected with *S. mutans* in a person with high caries prevalence than in a person with low prevalence.
5. Immunization of experimental animals against *S. mutans* reduces the incidence of dental caries.

6. Antimicrobial measures directed against *S. mutans* can dramatically reduce the incidence of dental caries.

The correlation between *S. mutans* and dental caries has been used for selection of children at a high risk to caries attack. Such children have obtained various preventive measures, and when the effect has been controlled by microbiological methods, a considerable caries reduction has been achieved. Some of the clinical studies which form a basis for the methods used in the individual case are described on page 85.

These studies clearly show that a strong correlation exists between *S. mutans* and dental caries. The reasons why this microorganism is cariogenic are not fully known, but it is most probably due to its unique combination of properties, listed below.

1. It colonizes the teeth.
2. It produces large amounts of extracellular polysaccharides that enable voluminous plaque formation.
3. It produces large amounts of acid even at low pH values.
4. It breaks down some salivary glycoproteins which might be of great importance for the initial development of carious lesions.

It should be noted, however, that although *S. mutans* has been strongly implicated in the development of caries, this does not mean that it is the *only* microorganism that causes caries nor does it mean that *S. mutans* is *always* cariogenic.

Lactobacilli

Lactobacilli can also be closely associated with caries, at least under special circumstances. The condition favoring these organisms is one where a mouth is subjected to a high and repeated intake of sugar between meals. Indeed, the number of lactobacilli in the oral cavity to a certain extent relates to the carbohydrate intake. Thus, the *Lactobacillus* count can be used both for an evaluation of the caries risk of the patient and for an assessment of the effect of dietary changes.

S. mutans and lactobacilli can be cultivated and identified readily. It is therefore possible to apply the knowledge now available about these microorganisms in the diagnosis treatment and prevention of dental caries. Where there is a high prevalence of *S. mutans* and lactobacilli in the plaque, there is generally a high number of these microorganisms in the saliva. For this reason, saliva samples (for example, paraffin-stimulated saliva) can be used routinely in examinations to evaluate the caries risk.

Actinomyces

In the last few years some species of *Actinomyces* bacteria, especially *Actinomyces viscosus,* have been associated with the development of root surface caries. *Actinomyces* strains are relatively poor acid producers. This means that they rarely induce enamel caries in experimental animals and that the development of root surface lesions is a comparatively slow process when these microorganisms are the causative factor. Selective media for cultivating *Actinomyces* in plaque and saliva samples have been developed but they are not yet used routinely. In patients with root surface caries, samples for cultivation of *S. mutans* and lactobacilli should be taken just as in cases of enamel caries. High numbers of these bacteria indicate that they are involved also in the development of caries lesions on the root surfaces; the treatment will then be the same as with enamel caries.

If, on the other hand, a person with root surface caries has low values of *S. mutans* and lactobacilli, sugar and refined carbohydrates are less important. Consequently, dietary counseling aimed at reducing the carbohydrate intake does not have to be given.

Diet

The importance of various dietary factors in the pathogenesis of caries has been discussed extensively elsewhere. Here, only the relationship between the microflora (especially *S. mutans* and lactobacilli) and carbohydrates (particularly sucrose) will be stressed.

Sucrose

The central role of sucrose for the development of dental caries is documented by a series of accurate observations. These include:

1. Studies of the history and the geographical variation in the prevalence of dental caries
2. Observations of isolated populations for which the environmental conditions have been changed
3. Clinical studies and clinical experiments
4. Observations of persons with hereditary fructose intolerance who cannot eat sucrose and who remain almost caries free on a Western-type diet
5. Experimental studies of animals
6. Studies of the relationship between *S. mutans* and caries

The Swedish Vipeholm study resolved a series of apparently contradictory observations. This study demonstrated conclusively that the *frequency* of sugar intake rather than the *total* sugar intake was of decisive importance in the development of caries. In this series of studies the importance of the concentration and the stickiness of the sugar product was also demonstrated. These factors influence the sugar elimination time, i.e., the time taken for elimination of sugar from the mouth after eating.

Starch is considerably less caries accelerating than sucrose. In animal experiments, monosaccharides such as glucose and fructose produce almost twice as much caries as starch. Sucrose causes roughly five times as much dental caries as starch, and in contrast to the monosaccharides and starch, sucrose also favors the development of smooth surface caries.

The reasons why sucrose has a much higher caries-inducing potential than other carbohydrates are:

1. Sucrose is a small uncharged molecule that easily diffuses into the dental plaque.
2. Sucrose is highly soluble and acts as a substrate both for production of extracellular polysaccharides and for acid production. Plaque bacteria produce acids at the same rate of speed from the disaccharide sucrose as from the monosaccharides glucose and fructose.
3. Sucrose favors the establishment of *S. mutans* on teeth, and a high sucrose intake gives rise to voluminous plaque formation.
4. Sucrose does not contain substances that can inhibit the plaque bacteria or form a protection on the enamel surface.

Sucrose is not required for the initial attachment of *S. mutans* to tooth surfaces. However, for further development of the microbial colony (i.e., for the intercellular adherence), sucrose plays a *key* role. With sucrose present *S. mutans* forms a sticky extracellular polysaccharide similar to dextran. This capacity allows *S. mutans* to form a firmly adherent colony on the tooth surface. Only with sucrose is such a sticky colony formed. Such a colony can be compared to a lens that concentrates the rays of the sun on a small point to cause a burn. The organisms in the center of the "bacterial lens" produce a carious lesion. The *S. mutans* colony also can be compared to road workers who, protected by a tent (polysaccharides) from rain (saliva), break up the surface of the street. By sometimes using a spade and sometimes a pneumatic drill, the workers dig a hole at various speeds. In the same way, different strains of *S. mutans* may make a hole in the tooth at different speeds because they have a varying virulence.

In addition to the capacities of *S. mutans* to produce large amounts of acids and extracellular polysaccharides, the ability to produce intracellular polysaccharides may be important for the virulence. These may serve as a substrate for acid production when the external supply of carbohydrates ceases. The intracellular polysaccharides therefore constitute the "between-meal snacks" for the streptococci. In animal experiments it has been shown that *S. mutans* strains that have lost their ability to produce intracellular polysaccharides have a lowered pathogenicity.

The facts that different strains of *S. mutans* can have a varying virulence and that the supply of carbohydrates from external sources can have different levels of importance serve to illustrate why caries risk cannot be assessed solely by determining the number of *S. mutans* or the frequency of sugar intake.

Host

One of the most important factors of the host that determines resistance to dental caries is the character and state of the tooth enamel. Return to the analogy about the road workers: The difficulty of their work depends on whether the street is paved or not and also on the ground conditions under the surface of the street.

It was believed that the resistance of the enamel to dissolution was considered of vital importance to the progress of caries. Lately, however, opinion has altered. The resistance of the tooth to caries is now thought to depend in part on whether it becomes colonized by cariogenic microorganisms. The composition of saliva and the nature of the film of glycoproteins deposited on the tooth surface, the pellicle, governs the establishment of the microflora on the tooth surface. It has not yet been determined what composition of salivary glycoproteins increases or decreases the caries risk.

Nonetheless, we can use the secretion rate and the buffering capacity of saliva to assess the caries risk. These saliva factors are, however, affected by a number of physiological and pathological conditions. In this context all the circumstances and facts that should be observed during the taking of case history and at the clinical examination will be fully outlined and discussed.

Effects on the main factors

Each of the three main factors in the development of caries—host, diet, and microflora—can be altered either separately or in combination. Genetic as well as environmental conditions can affect these factors. A variation in caries resistance may be due to both genetic and environmental conditions. In modern Western society, where caries-accelerating factors are very strong, genetic conditions seem to play a minor role.

Generally, the high prevalence of caries in the West is considered to be the result of caries-promoting dietary habits. As indicated by research findings during the last decade, however, the high prevalence may also be explained in another way; that is, highly virulent microorganisms may predominate in the Western world. Thus, the combination of virulent cariogenic microorganisms and a high and often repeated intake of sucrose results in a high caries risk. This combination is found in 10% to 20% of the Western population. The identification of these persons at high risk to caries is a problem of major importance, not only for the individuals concerned but also for the community.

When should the caries risk be assessed?

An assessment of the caries risk, which influences planning of therapy, selection of filling materials, and the date for recall examinations, forms the basis for various decisions in the everyday work of a dental practitioner. The assessment is generally based on only a clinical examination and a simple case history. The responsibility of the dentist is, however, to treat and prevent the disease rather than treat only the symptoms. When it is uncertain whether and how this can be achieved, the clinical examination and the case history should be supplemented. As a rule of thumb, completing examinations such as taking a dietary history and salivary and bacteriological samples should be performed for the following circumstances:

1. The caries picture is other than expected (for example, with regard to number, location, and appearance of the cavities).
2. Extensive restorative work is required and the previous caries activity has been high, or new surfaces with low caries resistance have been exposed (for example, root surfaces).
3. A high caries risk can be expected (for example, in connection with some general diseases or radically changed dietary habits and living conditions).

Examples of completing examinations

The following are actual patient cases that illustrate situations where full examination has been of value in the assessment of caries risk.

Case 1
Woman, 23 years old; almost caries free. She has visited the dentist once a year, and been examined regularly in the school dental service up to the age of 19. At a clinical examination four years later she exhibited large numbers of early approximal carious lesions. Salivary and microbiological examinations indicated that the caries risk was low.
Treatment: Only topical fluoride was applied; there were no fillings.
Control: At the clinical examinations one and two years later no new carious lesions were found. The results from objective tests confirmed that the caries risk continued to stay low.
Conclusion: The analysis prevented successive destruction of a good dentition by means of a restorative therapy that was not necessary.

Case 2
Man, 52 years old; extensive loss of teeth which for both functional and esthetical reasons requires attention. Salivary and microbiological examinations showed that the actual caries risk was low.

Treatment: The dentition was restored suitably with general oral hygiene instruction.
Control: After one and two years, there were no new lesions.
Conclusion: Both the dentist and the patient saved time and costs of caries preventive measures.

Case 3
Man, 45 years old; extensive loss of teeth (just as in case 2). Completing salivary and microbiological samples indicated a high caries risk.
Treatment: Before beginning the required bridgework measures were taken to reduce the caries risk. The effectiveness was assessed by new salivary and microbial analyses. When the caries risk was considered to be low the bridgework was completed.
Control: After one and two years, nothing remarkable.
Conclusion: In this case completing examinations and treatment of the cause of the disease itself prevented destruction of the expensive bridgework by secondary caries.

These three very typical cases illustrate how salivary and microbiological examinations can greatly assist the daily work of a dental practitioner. Such examinations, however, can also be used in the school dental service to identify children at a high caries risk for special preventive measures (see page 85).

Chapter 2

Case History and Clinical Examination

It is usual that before a patient is seen for the first time the dentist is provided with some personal data. Age and sex are important for assessment of the caries risk because the caries activity varies considerably in different age groups. Teeth are most susceptible to caries two to four years after eruption. Furthermore, the caries activity often increases when caries-susceptible root surfaces become exposed. Women generally have a higher caries prevalence than men.

Case history

The social background, birthplace and area where a person grows up, occupation, living conditions, and smoking and drinking habits all affect the dental as well as the general health and should be investigated and recorded. Such information is required to evaluate the caries status of the patient. It serves too as a guide for dentists when they have to decide on the most suitable preventive therapy and an indication for the level of cooperation that can be expected from the patient under treatment.

It is well known that social conditions and occupation can affect dietary habits and thereby the caries risk; for example, family stress, shift work, or drinking habits may increase the caries risk, although the latter are not so often considered. That is, a patient may drink sweet wine several times a day, another a hot toddy with sugar at night in order to fall asleep. It is also quite common for persons with alcohol problems to use mint drops to conceal alcoholic breath. Often such persons eat sweets to get "quick energy."

However busy a modern practitioner is, a true profile of the patient's life-style must be recorded. Only then can correct scientific treatment and prevention of dental disease be achieved. Many bonuses will accrue not only by the application of the science to the treatment but also by the increased confidence patients will gain by the ability to talk and become involved in the sensible control of the disease. In other words, the patient may alter his or her life-style for health benefits.

Many systemic diseases and their treatment may reduce the caries resistance of the patient, and when the balance is changed, caries-promoting factors may prevail. For example, most general diseases alter the salivary secretion rate causing it to go up or down. Psychiatric diseases and gastrointestinal disorders may also lead to frequent food nibbling, which of course increases the caries risk if the food contains sugar and starch.

Medication too can indirectly affect the caries activity through an anticholinergic effect. More than 100 medicines in use today presumably show as a side effect a reduction of the salivary secretion rate, therefore increasing the caries risk. In Table 3, various groups of diseases and corresponding medicines are listed which might reduce the salivary secretion rate.

Table 3 Groups of medicines with an inhibitory effect on the salivary secretion rate as a side effect

Diseases	Medication
Gastrointestinal disorders	Anticholinergics
Psychiatric diseases	Sedatives
Organic neurologic disorders	Neuroleptics
Allergic diseases	Antihistamines

Medicaments that contain sucrose can have a direct caries-promoting effect. Such medicines are cough drops, laxatives, antacids, and tonics. Lithium salts induce a heavy thirst which the patient often tries to overcome by drinking soft drinks.

The patient's chief complaint is an important part of the history and is generally disclosed at the first visit. A basic professional rule is that the patient should leave the office with his or her primary discomfort reduced.

Previous dental treatment—where, when, and how—is important to record. Dietary and oral hygiene habits, as well as earlier use of fluorides, also have to be noted.

The attitude of the patient to the teeth and to dental care will greatly influence decisions about the form and extension of therapeutic and preventive measures.

Clinical examination

The physical state often reveals some important clinical facts. Pregnancy, for example, can increase the caries risk because of the tendency to nibble, whereas obesity might be the result of a high and frequent sugar intake. Leanness, on the other hand, may be a consequence of anorexia nervosa; with this disease, a high caries activity is sometimes seen.

In addition to the physical state, the behavior and movements of the patient should also be observed. A reduced or impaired faculty of motion not only impairs cooperation with regard to oral hygiene, it may also have other effects. A reduced physical mobility may often affect dietary habits.

During intraoral examination, various facts should be observed. The most obvious are:

1. Conditions of the mucous membranes
2. Caries prevalence
3. Amount of plaque
4. Gingival and periodontal conditions
5. Localization and appearance of the carious lesions
6. Quality of previous dental care

A dry, dull mucosa might indicate a reduced salivary

secretion rate. The prevalence of caries is generally a good predictor for future caries risk. Plaque index and gingival index illustrate the ability and the interest of the patient to care for his or her teeth and therefore the behavior of the patient. The number and the localization of the carious lesions give information on the caries activity. If several cavities are found and if the lesions are soft and not pigmented, the caries activity may be high. Also the localization of the lesions can give important leads. Therapeutically, an initial lesion on the mesial surface of the first permanent molar in a 13-year-old differs from the same lesion in a 30-year-old. These examples are rather simple. It might be more complicated to determine the presence or absence of secondary caries underneath a full crown. It is often difficult to differentiate between a poor-fitting crown and secondary caries and often a radiograph is of little help. In patients such as these full examinations are essential.

In conclusion, it must be stressed that neither the case history nor the clinical examination is completely objective. Therefore, it might be difficult to assess the actual caries risk on these examinations alone. In such situations, salivary and microbiological examinations should also be used.

Radiographic examination

A combination of a clinical and a radiographic examination is the best method for the detection of as many carious lesions as possible. Radiographic examination is essential for detection of initial interproximal lesions and for the follow-up of their development.

However, high quality and standardization in the radiographic examination is essential. To achieve this the following points should be observed:

1. The darkroom work should be standardized.
2. The exposure should be done so that all surfaces of the actual teeth are reproduced with similar contrast.

Radiographic Examination

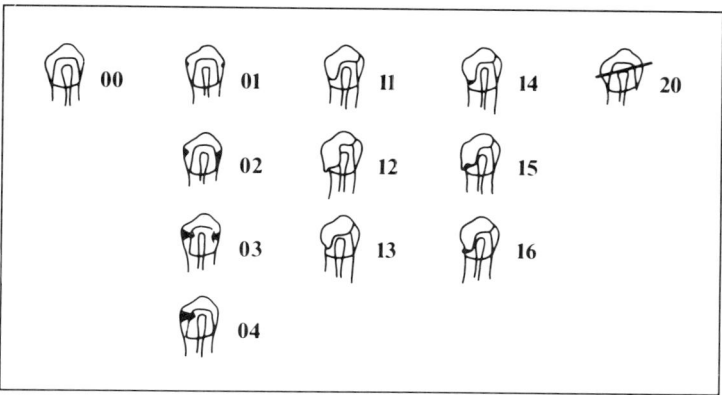

Fig. 3 System for recording the extension of carious lesions and the quality of restorations on radiographs (Gröndahl et al., 1977).

3. The projection angle should allow fully open interproximal contact.
4. The radiographs should be mounted as permanent records.
5. For examination and interpretation conditions such as lighting and magnification should be identical.
6. The results of the examination should be noted in writing.

A system for recording the extension of the carious lesions and the quality of the restorations has been developed (Fig. 3). With this system, a detailed picture of the actual status of the patient can be obtained and any changes between any two examinations can be noted in detail. In the individual case, it can therefore be decided more easily whether laboratory examinations have to be used in order to assess the actual caries risk.

Chapter 3

Dietary Analysis

As diet is one of the main factors in the development of dental caries, a dietary assessment is a fundamental part of the examination. It should always be done in patients with a high caries activity or in those with an unusual caries pattern.

In order to be able to give the patient correct information, the dentist not only has to know the dietary habits and social history of the patient, but also must have a fair knowledge of general nutrition. (Excellent texts on this subject are available and some of them are mentioned in the further reading list at the end of the book.)

Food intake and eating habits are among the most complex aspects of human behavior. Accurate assessment of nutrition needs and deficiencies is not easy. Although it is widely known that candies, cookies, and soft drinks can increase the caries risk, it is difficult to obtain reliable dietary data from the patient.

To determine food intake and food habits various techniques have been devised. One technique is to record the dietary intake during the preceding 24 hours, called the 24-hour recall. Another technique is to obtain a three- to seven-day written food record. The method used at the Department of Cariology at the University of Göteborg, Sweden, follows.

Recording dietary intake

The patient is asked to write down in detail everything he or she eats and drinks during three consecutive days. When,

Dietary Analysis

what, and how much of each food item was ingested should be recorded.

To clarify how detailed this dietary bookkeeping has to be done, show the patient an example of such a dietary recording (see below).

Example of a detailed dietary record

Day 1
November 20, 1984
- 7:15 a.m. 1 cup of coffee, 2 spoonfuls of sugar, cream, 2 pieces of toast with butter and honey.
- 9:15 a.m. 1 Lifesaver.
- 10:05 a.m. 1 cup of coffee, 2 spoonfuls of sugar, cream, 1 doughnut.
- 12:30 p.m. A hamburger on bun with onion, 1 slice of tomato, salad, a big portion of french fries; 1 glass of ice water; 1 cup of coffee, cream, and 2 spoonfuls of sugar.

etc.

It ought to be stressed that the dietary recording includes all medication and all small items such as lozenges and mints such as Lifesavers. The patient should therefore write down on a piece of paper whatever is placed in the mouth, the amount, and the time of consumption.

Evaluation of dietary history

In order to facilitate the evaluation of the food intake, different food guides are used. A popular food guide—for example, Canada's Food Guide (Fig. 4)—has four food groups: milk and milk products; meat, fish, and poultry; fruits and vegetables; and breads and cereals. The recommended number of servings and examples of one serving in each of the groups are shown in Fig. 5. The main nutrients in the various groups are:

Evaluation of Dietary History

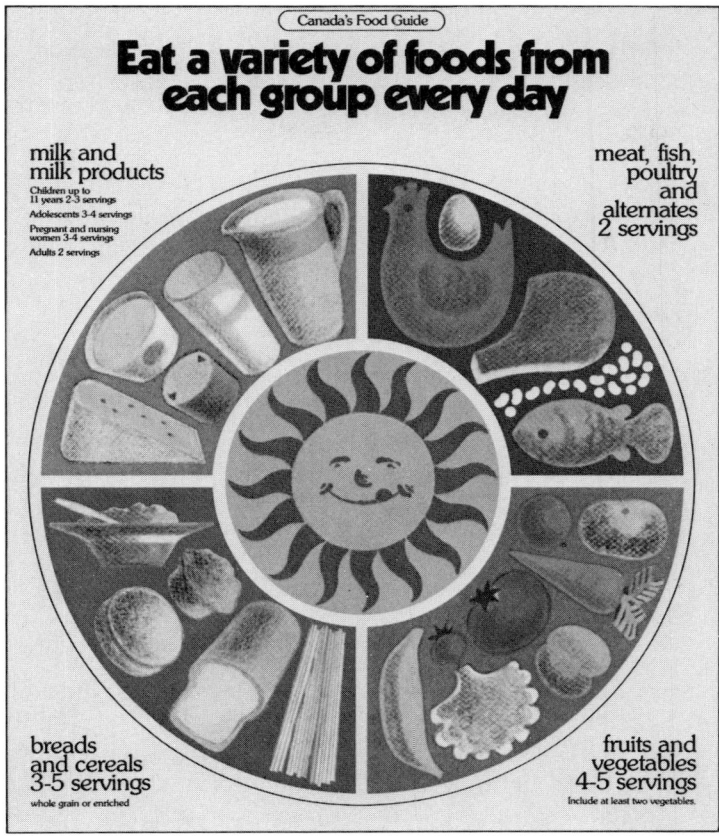

Fig. 4 Canada's Food Guide with the four food groups and the recommended number of servings. (From *Canada's Food Guide,* Health and Welfare Canada, 1983, reproduced with permission of the Minister of Supply and Services Canada.)

1. Milk and milk products: Protein, calcium, vitamins A and D, riboflavin
2. Meat, fish, and poultry: Protein, iron, vitamins A, D, B
3. Fruits and vegetables: Cellulose, pectin, minerals, carotene, iron and vitamin C
4. Breads and cereals: Carbohydrates, protein, iron, B vitamins

Diet Analysis
Use the chart below to record number of servings for each day

Food group	Suggested no. of daily servings (adults)	No. of servings Day 1	Day 2	Day 3	Portion considered for 1 serving
Milk and milk products	2*				1 cup† milk; 1½ oz. cheddar cheese
Meat, fish, poultry, and alternates	2				60–90 g (2–3 oz.) cooked lean meat, poultry or fish; 250 ml (1 cup) cooked dried peas, beans, or lentils
Fruits and vegetables	4–5				125 ml (½ cup) vegetables or fruits; 1 medium-sized potato, carrot, or tomato
Breads and cereals	3–5				1 slice of bread; 125 ml (½ cup) cooked cereal; 175 ml (3/4 cup) ready-to-eat cereal

*Adolescents and pregnant and nursing women: 3–4 servings.
†1 cup = 250 ml or 8 oz. (1 oz. = 28 g).

Fig. 5 Form for evaluation of the appropriate number of servings and examples of one serving in the different food groups.

When evaluating the dietary intake, a special form can be used (Fig. 5). The servings of each different food group are recorded, one mark for each serving, and the total intake for each day is compared with the recommended amount. A deficient intake is noted by circling the marks. For evaluation of the sucrose intake a separate form is used (Fig. 6). Sometimes it is valuable to ask the patient to circle all the foods on the dietary form that contain sucrose; this teaches where hidden sucrose can be found. Often the number of foods containing sucrose is considerably larger than anticipated by the patient.

Frequency of Sucrose Exposures			
	Day 1	Day 2	Day 3
At meals			
Between meals			
Total			

Fig. 6 Form for evaluation of the sucrose intake.

It should be stressed that the person who examines the record should have not only a basic knowledge in food composition and nutrition, but also the time and ability to obtain satisfactory information about the patient, including disease problems and the socioeconomic situation. These factors largely influence the food intake.

As stated earlier, food intake assessment is open to error. The patient knowing that sweets are bad for the teeth frequently will not admit a craving for them. For this reason, the dietary history in a caries-active patient should always be supplemented with a microbiological examination.

The *Lactobacillus* count, to a certain extent, reflects the total carbohydrate intake, whereas the *S. mutans* level primarily mirrors the sucrose consumption. An adolescent with no open carious lesions might, for example, have a high

Lactobacillus count not from eating sweets but from eating lots of bread. A patient with active carious lesions who has a low number of *S. mutans* and states that he or she has stopped eating sweets is probably telling the truth. These examples illustrate the value of determining both the *S. mutans* and the *Lactobacillus* count as a supplement to the dietary examination.

Chapter 4

Salivary Examination

Saliva affects the teeth and the microflora in different ways. Several components and properties of saliva have been associated with the development of dental caries. During the last few years, salivary factors influencing the colonization of cariogenic microorganisms on the teeth have been the focus of interest, but none of these have yet proved to be of diagnostic value. So far significant correlations have been found only between the salivary secretion rate and the buffer capacity on the one hand and the caries activity on the other. These important salivary properties can be assessed by means of simple methods.

Low salivary secretion rate and low buffer capacity lead to reduced elimination of microorganisms and food remnants, to impaired neutralization of acids, and to a reduced tendency to remineralization of early enamel lesions. A low salivary secretion rate is generally accompanied by an increased number of *S. mutans* and lactobacilli. Thus, an increased caries activity seen in persons with a reduced salivary secretion rate may be due not only to a reduced host resistance but also to an overwhelming microbial challenge.

Determination of salivary secretion rate

Material: Measuring cylinder, funnel, piece of paraffin wax (about 1.5 g), and a stopwatch.

Method: Have the patient hold the piece of paraffin wax in the mouth until it becomes soft; the saliva produced during

Salivary Examination

this time is swallowed. Start the stopwatch when the patient begins to chew on the wax. The saliva produced is expectorated with frequent intervals in the funnel and the measuring cylinder. After about five minutes the patient should stop chewing and expectorate the last portion of the stimulated saliva. When the salivary secretion rate is high, the time can be shortened. However, when the rate is low, it may have to be increased. As a rule, the patient should chew for at least two minutes, or 2 ml saliva should be collected. The volume of saliva secreted is measured and the secretion rate expressed in milliliters per minute (for example, 3.5 ml in five minutes is equal to 0.7 ml per minute).

Results: Normal secretion rate in adults: 1–2 ml per min
          Remarkably low secretion rate: <0.7 ml per min
          Xerostomia: <0.1 ml per min

A certain variation between two samples taken at different occasions is generally observed. To reduce this variation the samples should always be taken under as similar conditions as possible. The patient might be somewhat uneasy when the first sample is taken; this reduces the flow rate. The same effect is detected when the patient reads or is distracted in other ways. Therefore, when the saliva sample is taken, the patient should be left alone without any magazines, books, or other distractions. The saliva sample collected for determination of the secretion rate can be used also for determination of the buffer capacity and for microbiological examinations.

Buffer capacity

Material: Paraffin-stimulated saliva is obtained in the same way as previously described. As the buffer capacity of saliva generally increases after eating, the saliva samples for the determination should be taken about two hours after a meal.

Method: Add 3 ml of 0.005 NHCl to 1 ml of saliva. To eliminate carbon dioxide, shake the sample and remove the stopper. Let the sample stand for 10 minutes, and then measure the final pH. This can be done with pH indicator paper if a pH meter is not available. Special kits are commercially available (Dento-buff) that contain a small flask with a weak acid and a color indicator. The kit also holds a syringe with which 1 ml of the saliva sample can be injected into the test vial. After mixing, the resulting color is compared with an accompanying color chart.

Results: Normal buffer capacity: final pH between 5 and 7
          Low buffer capacity: final pH < 4

Values between pH 4 and 5 should be considered borderline values.

Discussion

The simplified methods using pH indicators may give results that are difficult to interpret at certain pH intervals. They are, however, sensitive and reliable enough for identification of patients with low buffer capacity. The methods, however, should not be used for differentiation between patients with normal and good buffer capacity.

As stated above, low salivary secretion rate and low buffer capacity may imply an increased caries risk. Because a reduced salivary secretion rate often is accompanied by increased numbers of *S. mutans* and lactobacilli a microbiological examination should be performed in such cases.

If the examination of the saliva shows that negative (low) values are present, it should be resolved whether they are occasional or constant. If they are constant the reason why has to be determined. Regarding measures for treating poor salivary values, see page 45.

Chapter 5

Microbiological Examination

Saliva sample

For determination of the level of *S. mutans* and *Lactobacillus* infection, it is most convenient to use a saliva sample.

The number of microorganisms in saliva varies at different times of the day. The samples should therefore be taken at the same time each day as much as possible—for example, at home in the morning, before toothbrushing, and before eating on the day the patient sees the dentist. If the sample is taken at the dental clinic, this should be done one to two hours after a meal.

Material: Material for sampling can be requested from a microbiological service laboratory where *S. mutans* and lactobacilli are cultivated routinely (in Canada, for example, from the Department of Oral Biology at the University of British Columbia). The materials needed are a piece of paraffin wax, a transport vial, a transport mailing tube, a form for necessary patient data, and a padded envelope. In addition, a 10 ml measuring cylinder and a funnel are useful (see chapter 4 for determination of the salivary secretion rate).

Method: Use paraffin-stimulated saliva. Ask the patient to chew on the paraffin wax for a few seconds. Do not collect the saliva obtained during this time because it often contains food remnants. Thereafter, have the patient chew on the paraffin wax using both sides of the mouth. The patient should expectorate the saliva into a measuring cylinder or a cup. Transfer the required amount to the transport vial, via a pipette or a syringe. Securely tighten the cap of the transport vial and turn it upside down or shake it in order to mix the

Microbiological Examination

transport fluid and the saliva. The name of the patient must be written on the label of the flask.

The same saliva sample can be used for determination of the salivary secretion rate, the buffer capacity, and the microbiological analysis.

A saliva sample might also be obtained without stimulation by chewing (e.g., when a large number of teeth is missing). Ask the patient to sit in a stooping position, let the saliva collect in the mouth, and expectorate into a beaker.

When the salivary secretion rate is strongly reduced (in xerostomia, for example), a sample can be obtained by having the patient rinse with 5 ml sterile water for one minute. The rinse is then expectorated and 1 ml transferred to the transport vial.

On the form sent to the laboratory, the type of sampling method used and the time of sampling have to be noted. It should also be explained what type of examination is required (number of *S. mutans* or lactobacilli, or both).

The sample should be kept in the refrigerator until it can be sent to the laboratory, which should be done in the fastest possible way. The saliva sample should never be allowed to sit in the mail over a weekend.

At the laboratory, the sample is homogenized, diluted, and cultivated on selective media for *S. mutans* and lactobacilli. In most laboratories, *S. mutans* is cultivated on mitis salivarius agar containing sucrose and bacitracin. For cultivation of lactobacilli generally SL-agar is used. The number of typical colonies at a suitable dilution is counted and the figure obtained is multiplied with the dilution factor. This gives the number of *S. mutans* and lactobacilli respectively for each milliliter of saliva.

High value: $>1,000,000$ *S. mutans,* $>100,000$ lactobacilli
Low value: $<100,000$ *S. mutans,* $<1,000$ lactobacilli

In a mouth rinse from xerostomia patients the number per milliliter of rinse is generally much lower than per milliliter of

Microbiological Examination

saliva. This must be accounted for when evaluating the effect of various preventive measures in such patients. It is better to use plaque samples (e.g., pooled plaque) and estimate the proportional distribution of *S. mutans* in xerostomia patients.

Plaque sample

In some cases an assessment of the frequency of *S. mutans* in plaque material can be of value. In addition to xerostomia patients, such cases include patients in whom the conditions on certain tooth surfaces are of interest (e.g., on exposed root surfaces with initial caries) or patients who have only a few teeth left and in whom extensive bridgework is being considered.

Method: Spray the teeth or tooth surface with water (plaque is microorganisms on teeth that cannot be removed by a stream of water). Keep the area free from saliva with cotton rolls and dry it slightly with compressed air. Dental plaque is collected by means of a wax carver, an excavator, or a scaler instrument. Transfer the sample to a vial containing 1 ml of transport fluid. If the number of microorganisms has to be assessed a standardized amount of plaque material can be collected by using a measuring spoon. Most laboratories send on request a small steel plate with an excavation taking 5 mg. This is filled with plaque material. The whole plate is then transferred to the small sample vial.

The laboratory generally gives the percentage of *S. mutans* in relation to the total number of streptococci in the plaque material. For an assessment of the result, the following information can be of value:

High value: $>10\%$ *S. mutans*
Low value: $<1\%$ *S. mutans*

A significant correlation is found between the salivary concentration of *S. mutans* and its proportion in dental

Microbiological Examination

plaque. When more than 1% of the total strep in plaque material are *S. mutans,* the mean value per milliliter of saliva is more than 1,000,000. Less than 0.3% generally corresponds to less than 300,000 per milliliter of saliva.

Chapter 6

Assessment of Findings

For assessment of the actual caries risk, facts from the case history, the clinical and radiographic examination, the dietary history, and the supplementary laboratory examinations all have to be considered.

No single negative factor implies a high caries risk. Both the sucrose consumption and the number of *S. mutans* are closely associated with dental caries, but many persons have high numbers of *S. mutans* without developing caries. Likewise there are persons who eat sucrose frequently but are caries free.

These examples illustrate that the development of caries would better fit the following equation: *S. mutans* × sucrose = dental caries. But dental caries cannot be expressed in absolute mathematical terms. Some persons have only a few small lesions, whereas others develop a large number of cavities. The difference might be due to different magnitude of the caries-inducing factors: *S. mutans* and sucrose. Table 4 illustrates this principle.

Table 4 also illustrates that even if two caries-inducing factors have different magnitudes the end product can be the

Table 4 Equation with examples resulting in different or same amount of dental caries

S. mutans	×	Sucrose	=	Dental caries
2		2		4
10		10		100
10		1		10
1		10		10

Assessment of Findings

same. As mentioned previously, various strains of *S. mutans* might have different virulence. Therefore, the same number of organisms per milliliter of saliva may imply quite a different caries risk. In addition to caries-inducing factors having different magnitudes, varying host resistance complicates the assessment of the caries risk. It must be remembered that dental caries is a multifactorial disease.

Some of the factors involved can be illustrated in the following formula:

S. mutans $\times$ lactobacilli $\times$ sucrose $\times$ salivary secretion rate $\times$ salivary buffer capacity $\times$ fluoride supplement $\times$ tooth resistance $\times$ general diseases $\times$ medication $\times$ socioeconomic factors $\times$ other factors $= ?$

As the magnitude of many of the factors is difficult to assess, it is obvious that the size of the final product cannot be determined exactly.

A practical way to assess the actual caries risk is illustrated in Table 5. In this table the different facts that can be used in the assessment have been distributed among the three main factors of host, diet, and microflora. Some of them can be recorded objectively, e.g., number of *S. mutans* and lactobacilli, the salivary secretion rate, and the buffer capacity of the saliva. Other factors such as fluoride supplement and sucrose consumption have to be estimated. The more objective the data is, the more reliable is the assessment. Simultaneous occurrence of a series of negative factors increases the probability of a high risk.

If case history and current state indicate a high actual caries risk and supplementary laboratory examinations support the assumption, it is not enough merely to accept the observation. To treat only the symptoms by filling the cavities is a wrong and incomplete approach. It is the disease itself that has to be treated. Therefore, a low salivary secretion rate, for example, should be increased or a high number of *S. mutans* should be reduced. The effect of the measures taken should then be checked in an objective way.

Table 5 Evaluation of the caries risk*

	Positive factors	Negative factors
Host		
General	Good health	Systemic diseases, e.g., gastric ulcer or allergy
	No medication	Medication with saliva-affecting drugs or medicines containing sugar
Social factors	Regular working hours	Shift work, stress
Teeth	Fluoride supplementation DMFT low	No fluorides DMFT high
	Carious lesions on surfaces at risk	Carious lesions on surfaces not normally affected
	Carious lesions hard, pigmented	Carious lesions soft, whitish appearance
Saliva	Normal secretion rate and buffer capacity	Low secretion rate and buffer capacity
Diet		
General	Well balanced	Deficient intake
Sucrose	Low intake especially between meals	Frequent intake of caries-accelerating snacks
Microflora		
	Low numbers of *S. mutans* and lactobacilli	High numbers of *S. mutans* and lactobacilli
	Good oral hygiene	Large amounts of plaque

*The caries risk describes to what extent a person at a particular time runs the risk of developing carious lesions. It is expressed as high, low, or levels in between.
The more objective the data the more reliable the assessment. Simultaneous occurrence of many negative factors increases the probability of a high risk.

Chapter 7

Managing Dietary Problems

The dietary factor that primarily increases the caries risk is frequent intake of sucrose in sticky form between meals. Dietary counseling, therefore, must deal with the between-meal eating of sugar. In order to obtain a good result, it is necessary to teach the patient to eat a nutritionally adequate diet on which he or she can feel satisfied from one meal to the next one. Dietary recommendations to persons of different ages are described in the food guide (see Fig. 4). Here, the emphasis will be focused on the counseling of adults with a high caries risk.

Dietary information

Recommendations about good nutrition are available in the form of dietary guidelines and food guides from health authorities in various countries. Such material should be used for general information.

Special information about diet and dental caries is available from both the Canadian and American Dental Association. Call the patient's attention to the following facts:

1. Frequent intake of sucrose is the most important caries-inducing dietary factor.
2. The composition of meals determines the state of satiety and thereby affects the need for between-meal nibbling.

Dietary counseling

Dietary counseling must be adjusted not only to the patient's dietary history but also to the case history and to observations made at the clinical and laboratory examinations. Remember: a diet that does not imply any caries risk for a person with a normal salivary secretion rate might be caries conducive in an individual with a low salivary secretion rate. If it is necessary to change the dietary habits more drastically it is valuable to know about the physiological mechanisms that govern hunger and satiety. A patient might, for example, reveal functional symptoms of hypoglycemia such as restlessness and irritability when a frequent carbohydrate intake is replaced by a protein-rich diet eaten only at the ordinary meals. In order to give the patient appropriate and motivating instructions, more than nutritional knowledge is required. Consequently, if dietary counseling is given by an auxiliary, the main points should be reinforced by the dentist.

Generally, it is convenient to start with the patient's dietary history. Suggest certain changes in agreement with the patient, and give the patient reasonable and realistic recommendations. The extent to which these are adjusted must relate to both the practicality and compliance of the patient.

The *goal* of the individual dietary counseling is to starve the acid-producing microorganisms in the oral cavity by a reduced intake of sugar and refined carbohydrates. In order to achieve this goal, it is necessary to change the main meals in such a way that the need for between-meal eating is reduced.

Advise the patient to:

1. Eliminate sucrose-containing between-meal snacks and avoid sugar in coffee and tea. Suggest alternative between-meal consumption that does not contain sugar. Tell the patient that eating fruits should be confined to mealtime.
2. To decrease sucrose consumption as much as possible, call the patient's attention to foods with high concentrations of hidden sucrose, e.g., ketchup, mustard, breakfast cereals, fruit drinks, and fruit yogurts.

    Do not recommend unlimited substitution by sorbitol

Dietary Recommendations
Breakfast:_____
Lunch:_____
Between meals:_____
Dinner:_____
Definitely avoid eating:_____
Eat more:_____
Good luck!
Signature:_____

Fig. 7 Form for dietary recommendations.

sweetened products. *S. mutans* and lactobacilli ferment this sugar alcohol and increased proportions of *S. mutans* and lactobacilli have been found in plaque material from persons who have used sorbitol regularly for a couple of months.

If the measures above have not been efficient, carbohydrate restriction during a short period of time (Jay, 1947) can be tried. To reduce the total carbohydrate intake to 100 g per day is difficult, however. This method, therefore, should be confined to patients with a pronounced "craving for sweets." This craving can be overcome in one to two weeks if the patient strictly adheres to a diet with a very low carbohydrate content.

The individual recommendations should be given to the patient in writing (Fig. 7). Keep a copy of the recommendations with the patient's records.

Discussion

Food intake and dietary habits are very difficult to influence. To find out whether the patient has followed the suggested dietary recommendations the dentist can simply ask the patient about any changes. However, it is much better to complete a follow-up microbiological examination. If the patient drastically changes his or her dietary habits and refrains from a high and repeated sucrose intake, high *S. mutans* and *Lactobacillus* counts should be reduced to about 10% of the original value within two weeks.

If the microbiological examination does not reveal the desired result, it is probable that the patient has not followed the recommendations. The patient might eat food with a high amount of hidden sucrose or, in another case, she or he might eat a lot of fruit. Therefore, it might be expedient to ask the patient to make a new recording of food intake.

The actual patient records in Table 6 illustrate the effect of different types of dietary recommendations on the *Lactobacillus* and *S. mutans* count (see also cases 2 and 3 on pages 76 and 77).

Table 6 Effect of dietary recommendations on lactobacilli and *S. mutans* in different patients

Patient	Day	Lactobacilli	*S. mutans*	Recommendations
		per ml saliva		
A.B., secretary, 25 years old	1	700,000	1,600,000	Eliminate sucrose-containing between-meal snacks
	30	51,000	230,000	
M.A., housewife, 36 years old	1	8,800,000	4,500,000	Refrain from sucrose and refined carbohydrates
	240	64,000	180,000	
	450	46,000	210,000	
H.B., taxi driver, 30 years old	1	390,000		Refrain from sugar in coffee and tea and on breakfast cereals
	100	5,700		
	250	9,700		
	310	10,000		

Summary

The basic principles for dietary counseling are as follows:

1. Start with the patient's dietary history.
2. Suggest changes of the main meals in such a way that the need for between-meal eating is reduced.
3. Give the patient reasonable and realistic recommendations.
4. Eliminate sucrose-containing between-meal snacks. Call the patient's attention to foods with hidden sugar.

Chapter 8

Treating Poor Salivary Values

Low salivary secretion rate and low buffer capacity may imply an increased caries risk. It is important, therefore, to try to change salivary conditions. The ways by which the salivary secretion rate can be influenced, however, are limited. Fairly simple measures might have an effect. An increased salivary secretion rate is generally accompanied by an increased buffer capacity.

Measures

1. Try to find the cause of the low salivary secretion rate. If necessary get in touch with the patient's physician. If the patient takes medicine with a side effect that reduces the salivary secretion rate, ask the physician if an alternative medication is feasible. A case in which the cause of a low salivary secretion rate has not been diagnosed should be referred to a physician for analysis and for radiologic examination. The cause of a low secretion rate should be remedied, if possible.

2. Recommend a diet that requires chewing and that has a high content of protein and vegetables. Such a diet generally leads to an increased salivary secretion rate and increased buffer capacity. In cases with a low salivary secretion rate the protective effect of topical fluorides should be utilized as much as possible. Furthermore, the importance of a rigorous oral hygiene should be stressed. Persons with a reduced salivary secretion rate often start to use sugar-containing lozenges spontaneously. From a caries point of view, this can

lead to disastrous consequences. Also, sorbitol-containing sweets might increase the caries risk as both lactobacilli and *S. mutans* ferment this sugar alcohol, and these microorganisms show a proportional increase when the saliva secretion rate is reduced. These facts and the possible caries-inducing risk of the frequent use of sorbitol should therefore be mentioned.

3. If no organic background to a reduced salivary secretion rate is found, the following methods can be used in order to obtain an increased salivary flow:

- Chewing on paraffin wax: A piece of paraffin wax (about 1.5 g) is chewed on both sides of the mouth three to five times a day. Paraffin wax with a melting point of 42°C should be used; convenient-size pieces can be made by pouring melted paraffin in aluminum candy cups.

- Calcium phosphate tablets. *Recipe:*

Xylitol	1.28 g
Citric acid	28 mg
Maleic acid	56 mg
Tricalciumphosphate	28 mg
Magnesium stearate	85 mg
Collodium	8 mg

    Mix above ingredients into one tablet. Suck on tablet three to five times per day for two to three weeks.

- Nicotinamide: 0.1 g in gelatin capsules, 3 capsules per day for 2-3 weeks

These various methods and tablets have been tried for several years at the cariology clinic in Göteborg in patients with a reduced salivary secretion rate. All of these methods have given substantial relief of dryness of the mouth. The volumes of saliva have also increased markedly. Whatever measures are taken to increase flow, objective methods should be instituted to check if the salivary secretion rate increases.

4. If a low salivary secretion rate still cannot be increased, conventional preventive measures have to be intensified by the following:

- **Rigorous** plaque control. Professional tooth cleaning two times per month.
- Topical fluoride application aiming at an increase of fluoride in the outermost part of the enamel and exposed root surfaces. A practical method is the use of fluoride gel in custom-fitted vinyl applicators (see page 65). Another method that might be of value is the use of fluoride varnish.
- Analysis of the microflora and—if necessary—antimicrobial measures (see page 63).

5. To relieve some of the discomfort of xerostomia "artificial saliva" might be used. *Recipe:*

Sodium carboxymethylcellulose	1 g
Xylitol solution (70%)	4.3 g
Potassium chloride	0.1 g
Sodium chloride	0.1 g
Sodium fluoride	0.2 mg
Magnesium chloride	5 mg
Calcium chloride	15 mg
Potassium phosphate	40 mg
Potassium sulfocyanide	10 mg
Methyl para oxibenz	0.1 g
Distilled water	ad 100 g

The effect of various measures on salivary secretion rate and buffer capacity is illustrated in Table 7 from some actual patient records.

Table 7 Effect of various measures on salivary secretion rate and buffer capacity

Patient	Day	Secretion rate (ml/min)	Buffer capacity (pH)	Measures
F.A., 23 years old, poor diet	0 450	1.06 1.7	4.2 6.1	Improvement of diet, filling of teeth
K.M., 56 years old, root surface caries	0 415	0.6 1.1	3.7 7.2	Improvement of diet, acid phosphate tablets
H. S., 30 years old, irradiation against head and neck	0 120 440 720	0.1 0.44 0.85 1.33	— — — —	Chewing on paraffin wax

Summary

The basic principles to follow in patients with poor salivary values are:

1. Try to find the cause of the low salivary secretion rate. Get in touch with the patient's physician if necessary.
2. Recommend a diet that requires chewing and that has a high content of protein and vegetables.
3. If no organic background to the reduced secretion rate is found, recommend that the patient chew on paraffin wax, or take saliva stimulating tablets or Nicotinamide. Check the effect by new saliva samples.
4. Institute strict preventive measures.
5. In severe cases prescribe the use of "artificial saliva."

Chapter 9

Reducing Cariogenic Microorganisms

Some microorganisms are of greater importance than others for the development of dental caries. Treatment of the cause of the disease therefore requires a microbiological examination.

If high numbers of *S. mutans* and lactobacilli have been found, these numbers have to be reduced. This can be accomplished by various measures, described below. The effect of the treatment is reinforced with the help of a new microbiological examination.

As caries activity is due to a variety of factors and not only to the number of cariogenic bacteria, no absolute numbers can be given for the microbial count reduction in individual cases. For guidance, however, the following values are used:

S. mutans: < 100,000 per ml saliva
Lactobacilli: < 10,000 per ml saliva

If the number of *S. mutans* is lower than 100,000 per milliliter of saliva, generally only a few teeth are colonized by these microorganisms. In group studies, less than 250,000 *S. mutans* and 10,000 lactobacilli per milliliter of saliva have been associated with a low caries activity.

When high numbers of *S. mutans* and lactobacilli have been detected, the following measures should be taken (for effects of different measures, see Table 8).

Table 8 Effect of different measures on the number of *S. mutans* and lactobacilli

Patient	Day	*S. mutans*	Lactobacilli	Measures
		—per ml saliva—		
A. A., housewife, 35 years old	0	2,500,000	1,700,000	Dietary changes and restorations
	75	900,000	140,000	
	405	200,000	80,000	
L. J., student, 20 years old	0	3,500,000	430,000	Carbohydrate restriction
	21	100,000	25,000	
	28	0	20,000	
	84	0	20,000	
C. P., secretary, 29 years old	0	1,500,000	4,100,000	Chlorhexidine gel, elimination of lozenges
	24	20,000	59,000	

Mechanical measures

1. Carious lesions are filled (temporary material can be used) and faulty fillings are treated.
2. Overhangings and underfillings, as well as unanatomical interproximal areas, are adjusted.
3. Fissures are sealed in newly erupted teeth.
4. Oral hygiene instruction is given.

These measures generally give a certain reduction of the number of both *S. mutans* and lactobacilli. Sometimes, however, the effect is small; therefore, such approaches cannot be relied on alone.

Dietary measures

This treatment starves the acid-producing microorganisms and increases the proportional distribution of nonaciduric and acidogenic bacteria. This effect can be obtained by:

Reducing Cariogenic Microorganisms

1. Avoiding sucrose-containing foods and snacks between meals.
2. Substituting sucrose-containing foods (lozenges, chewing gum) with foods containing artificial sweeteners such as xylitol. Remember not to recommend sorbitol-containing products as this sugar alcohol is fermented by *S. mutans* and lactobacilli.
3. Restricting carbohydrates, i.e., reducing the total daily carbohydrate intake to 100 g during a two-week period.

Both *S. mutans* and lactobacilli are affected by dietary measures. By elimination of sucrose the number of *S. mutans* is generally reduced. In order to obtain a reduction of the *Lactobacillus* count, the total carbohydrate intake as a rule also has to be reduced. In young people, for example, who need a lot of energy, the continuous eating of bread has to be substituted by a protein-rich between-meal snack. The more strict the reduction of the refined carbohydrates, the more rapid is the change of the microflora. A two-week carbohydrate restriction should reduce the *Lactobacillus* count to about 10% of the original value providing retention areas such as open cavities have been eliminated. If the dietary changes are less drastic it will take two to three months before a definite change of the microflora can be observed.

In highly motivated patients, a clear-cut reduction of the number of *S. mutans* and lactobacilli is achieved in two patients out of three. In the remaining cases, additional measures have to be taken (see below).

Chemical and antimicrobial measures

These procedures aim to reduce the ability of bacteria to adhere to the tooth surface or to eliminate the cariogenic bacteria. Fluoride, still the most effective chemotherapeutic substance against dental caries, can be used to achieve both goals. To obtain an antimicrobial effect, fluoride solutions or fluoride gel in vinyl applicators can be used (see chapter 10).

Reducing Cariogenic Microorganisms

When using vinyl applicators, custom-fitted models, because they leak less than ready-mades, are generally preferred. This is important for preventing the ingestion of large amounts of fluoride. Using various methods and materials the dentist can produce different types of applicators.

For treatment with fluoride gel 1% sodium fluoride or 1.2% acidulated phosphate fluoride (APF) gels can be used in adults for intensive treatment during a period of two to three weeks. Due to the risk of toxic effects, 1% fluoride gels should not be used in small children (see page 73). In adults, 0.2% fluoride gels can be used routinely for a longer period of time.

S. mutans is considerably more sensitive to chlorhexidine than are other streptococci colonizing the tooth surface, for example, *Streptococcus sanguis*. Treatment with chlorhexidine gel therefore results in elimination of, or reduction of, the number of *S. mutans* concomitant with a proportional increase of the noncariogenic *S. sanguis*. Chlorhexidine is an excellent aid which should be used when other measures have not given a desired effect. Brushing the teeth with a chlorhexidine solution or a chlorhexidine gel has much less effect on *S. mutans* than chlorhexidine gel treatment, and this is therefore preferred. It is also advantageous to confine the antimicrobial treatment to the site of infection, as *S. mutans* mainly colonizes the teeth. Brushing also affects the bacteria on the tongue and the mucous membranes.

When using the vinyl applicators, five to 10 drops of the gel should be evenly spread and the patient should be encouraged to chew a little on the trays in order to press the gel into interproximal areas. The applicators should be used five minutes per day for two weeks. If the patient does not cooperate, the gel treatment can be given in the dental office. Then, the patient is treated at three five-minute sessions for two consecutive days the third week. Between each five-minute application the patient should rinse with water.

The effect on the microflora should be checked by a microbiological examination. When the desired result has been achieved, the chlorhexidine gel can be substituted with fluoride gel or fluoride rinsing. If the number of *S. mutans* has not been drastically reduced, the patient probably has not used the gel as prescribed.

In patients with a large number of chalky enamel lesions or root surface caries, a combined chlorhexidine-fluoride gel can be used. However, as chlorhexidine only needs to be used during a short period of time in order to reduce the *S. mutans* infection, it is generally preferable to use the two substances separately.

Summary

The basic principles to follow for reducing the number of cariogenic microorganisms:

1. Eliminate retention areas and institute good oral hygiene.
2. Recommend reduced intake of sugar and refined carbohydrate in order to starve the acid-producing microorganisms.
3. Check the effect by microbiological examinations.
4. If a satisfactory reduction of cariogenic microorganisms has not been obtained by the above measures use topical application of stannous fluoride or chlorhexidine gel in vinyl applicators.

Chapter 10

Fluoride Prevention in Adults

Fluorides have a caries preventive effect not only in children but also in adults. Newly exposed root surfaces are just as easily decayed as newly erupted teeth. Consequently, the caries preventive effect of fluorides should also be utilized in adults. It is not only chalky enamel lesions that can be stopped by topical fluoride application but also early carious lesions on root surfaces. A general principle to remember is that the higher the caries risk, the more intensive the fluoride treatment should be.

Mechanisms of action

1. Fluoride reduces the solubility of enamel and dentin in acids; nonvital teeth are also affected. F ions might substitute OH ions in the hydroxyapatite; this reaction decreases the solubility.
2. Fluoride increases the tendency of early enamel and dentinal carious lesions to remineralize. At the same calcium and phosphate concentration and at the same pH, the tendency of calcium phosphates to reprecipitate on the tooth surfaces increases if fluoride is present.
3. Fluoride decreases the surface energy of the tooth substance. As a consequence, the ability of microorganisms to adhere to the tooth is reduced.
4. Fluoride has an antienzymatic and an antimicrobial effect. At higher concentrations, fluoride solutions can have a bactericidal effect. At the fluoride concentrations,

which are found in plaque material after fluoride rinsing, an antienzymatic effect can be expected. Thus, the plaque bacteria's capacity for acid production may be reduced, and the production of extracellular polysaccharides may be inhibited. Finally, fluoride can reduce the synthesis of intracellular polysaccharides, i.e., the buildup of a reserve supply for acid production in *S. mutans*.

The effect of fluoride depends on:

1. The type of fluoride compound used (For example, SnF_2 has a much stronger bactericidal effect than does NaF.)
2. The concentration of the fluoride solution
3. The pH of the fluoride solution
4. The duration of the application
5. How frequently the fluoride solution is applied
6. The sensitivity of the microorganisms

Various methods of topical fluoride application

Fluoride-containing dentifrices

Fluoride-containing dentifrices characterized as the cornerstones in caries prevention, should be used as basic prevention in all patients.

Fluoride mouth rinses

For daily use, 0.025% or 0.05% NaF solution is recommended. For rinsing once a week, 0.2% NaF solution should be used. Daily rinsing is preferred.

If an antimicrobial effect on *S. mutans* is desired, 0.4% SnF_2 solution can be used according to the following prescription:

Stannous fluoride 1 g
Glycerol (free from water) 250 g
7.5 ml of the SnF_2 solution is mixed before use with 7.5 ml of water and divided in three portions of 5 ml for mouth rinsing according to the following schedule:
1. 5 ml 15 sec, expectorate
2. 5 ml 1 min, expectorate
3. 5 ml 1 min, expectorate

This treatment is repeated daily for two weeks. After this period new microbial samples are taken (for illustration of the effect, see case 5, page 81). SnF_2 solutions might stain early enamel lesions. If such areas are treated with NaF before the use of SnF_2, the risk of discoloration is reduced.

Fluoride tablets

Fluoride tablets can be used as a basis for prevention in patients who cannot use fluoride-containing dentifrices. They can also be used instead of mouth rinses in patients who are unable to rinse (e.g., some handicapped persons). Chewing on a tablet containing 0.25 mg F gives a fluoride concentration of about 200 ppm in the saliva.

Fluoride solutions professionally applied

A 2% NaF solution is generally applied three to four times with an interval of one week between the applications. As an alternative, an 8% SnF_2 solution can be used. *Recipe:*

0.8 g SnF_2
Lactose q.s., in gelatine capsules: 100

The content of one capsule is dissolved in 10 ml distilled water immediately before use. The 8% solution remains active for about 20 minutes and should then be discarded. A new solution should be made up for each patient.
The SnF_2 solution has a strong bactericidal effect and

topical application generally results in a reduction of the number of *S. mutans* and a reduced tendency to plaque formation. To avoid staining of chalky enamel lesions, such areas of the teeth should be treated with NaF solutions or fluoride varnish before treatment with SnF_2.

Fluoride-containing varnish

As an alternative to professionally-applied fluoride solutions, fluoride-containing varnish can be used (e.g., Duraphat). One milliliter of Duraphat contains 23 mg fluoride, which corresponds to about 100 fluoride tablets. In view of the high fluoride concentration, the application of varnish should be confined to only those tooth surfaces that actually need protection. In an adult with 28 teeth, about 0.5 ml varnish is required. Treatment with varnish should be repeated four times a year in persons with a high caries risk, on chalky enamel lesions, and on root surfaces with beginning decay.

After final polishing of new fillings, fluoride solution or fluoride varnish should be applied to restore the high content of fluoride in the outermost part of the tooth enamel that may have been removed during polishing.

The use of fluoride-containing varnish does not significantly reduce the number of *S. mutans* in plaque and saliva.

Fluoride-containing polishing pastes

When the teeth are polished, part of the fluoride-rich outer enamel surface is removed. In order to compensate for loss, polishing pastes containing fluoride should be used. Suitable pastes with varying polishing effects are available. They contain NaF or Na_2PO_3F and a compatible polishing substance.

Fluoride gels

In patients with a high caries risk, fluoride-containing gels should be used. High-risk patients are those who have received irradiation to the head and neck, or are receiving medication and therefore have a low salivary secretion rate.

Depending on the evaluation of the caries risk, either a 0.2 or a 1% fluoride gel is used. The patient can apply the gel at home. Custom-fitted, individually made vinyl applicators allow for smaller amounts of gel to be used. This is important because swallowing the gel might imply risk for toxic effects. For this reason, gels sold over the counter in the United States should contain no more than 120 mg of fluoride and should be packaged in containers with child-resistant closures.

Indications

In persons with a low caries risk the use of a fluoride-containing dentrifice is sufficient. With an increasing caries risk the fluoride treatment should be intensified and, depending on need and compliance, the following steps can be recommended:

1. Daily mouth rinsing or using fluoride tablets
2. Professionally applied fluoride solution or fluoride varnish
3. Treatment with fluoride gel

Controls

Just as other treatment procedures that increase resistance against or reduce the cause of the disease, the effect of fluoride treatment has to be checked. This can be done in the following ways:

1. Record the symptoms from sensitive cervical margins of teeth.
2. Record the appearance of chalky enamel lesions. A

detailed note about the appearance and surface texture of the initial carious lesion is put into the patient's record. The patient is informed that the rough surfaces will disappear if the recommendations given are followed. At the next visit the lesion's appearance is compared with the notation in the record. Important: Do not forget to praise the patient if a good result—remineralization—has taken place.
3. Examine the number of *S. mutans* in the saliva. After using an SnF_2 mouth rinse according to the recommendations, a considerable drop in the *S. mutans* count should be evident.

Summary

The basic principles for fluoride treatment in adults are:

1. The higher the caries risk, the more intensive the fluoride treatment should be.
2. If possible, fluorides should be applied frequently.
3. The type of administration should be adjusted to the patient's ability to comply.
4. The effect of the treatment should always be checked.

Chapter 11

Principles of Treatment: Case Studies

The prerequisite for adequate treatment is a correct diagnosis. The diagnosis should include an assessment of the actual caries risk. If the caries risk is low, the treatment can be confined to symptomatic measures, i.e., to restoration of the carious lesions.

If it is not certain that the caries risk is low, symptomatic treatment is given and the patient is recalled three to six months later. At this occasion, the clinical examination is again supplemented with an analysis of salivary and microbial conditions.

When the caries risk is considered high, the cause of the disease should be *taken care of* before a permanent rehabilitation is performed. The measures taken depend on the results of the laboratory examinations. The patient should not be burdened with treatment that is not indicated. It is, however, extremely important that the effect of the treatment of the cause of the disease is controlled by means of objective methods. The data obtained form a basis for the final planning of the restorative treatment.

On the following pages, the principles for treatment are illustrated. Six patient cases are described. The first demonstrates that the dentist can save time and costs for himself or herself and the patient by simple salivary and microbiological examinations. Without such a test, he or she would have to spend a lot of time on preventive measures not indicated. Cases 2 to 5 illustrate the principles for treatment of the cause of the disease, which are used at the Department of Cariology at the University of Göteborg. The sixth and last case has been included in order to demonstrate that dental caries can be caused by specific microorganisms, not only in animals but also in humans.

Principles of Treatment: Case Studies

Case 1

I. B., woman, 28 years old with phobia of dental treatment.
From the case history: No visits to a dentist for 10 years. Two children. Ate lots of sweets during her pregnancies. Now avoids sucrose because eating sugar causes toothaches.
Clinical examination: About 25 large cavities, some of which are heavily pigmented and have a hard bottom (see Figs. 9a and b in color atlas).
Dietary history: No nutritional deficiencies, low sucrose intake.

Laboratory examinations:

Day	Secretion rate, ml/min	Buffer capacity, pH	*S. mutans/* ml saliva	Lactobacilli/ ml saliva
1	1.0	3.5	38,000	18,000

Low numbers of *S. mutans* and lactobacilli supported the case history as well as the dietary history.
Treatment: The cavities were restored (see Figs. 9c and d in color atlas). No preventive measures were instituted. No new carious lesions after one and two years, respectively.

Case 2

M. L., woman, 30 years old.
From the case history: Housewife, two children. Has been treated with psychopharmaca because of depression. Complains of feeling occasional dryness in the mouth.
Clinical examination: Chalky enamel lesions; cavities encircle the tooth neck on some teeth (see Figs. 10a to c in color atlas).
Dietary history: Diet deficient with regard to fruits and vegetables. Sugar in coffee and tea. Eats lots of bread.

Laboratory examinations:

Month	Secretion rate, ml/min	Buffer capacity, pH	*S. mutans/* ml saliva	Lactobacilli/ ml saliva
1	0.5	4.3	2,500,000	1,200,000

Principles of Treatment: Case Studies

Treatment: Temporary fillings; daily fluoride mouth rinses (0.05% NaF); chewing on paraffin wax in order to stimulate the secretion of saliva.
Dietary counseling: Increase the intake of fruits and vegetables; refrain from sugar in coffee and tea.

Month	Secretion rate, ml/min	Buffer capacity, pH	S. mutans/ ml saliva	Lactobacilli/ ml saliva
2	1.2	4.3	<100	115,000

Definite increase of the salivary secretion rate and reduction of the number of *S. mutans* and lactobacilli.
Restorations: Amalgam and composite fillings.
At the control examination one year later, the following data were obtained:

Month	Secretion rate, ml/min	Buffer capacity, pH	S. mutans/ ml saliva	Lactobacilli/ ml saliva
14	1.3	5.2	200,000	< 100

Conclusion: In this case, information and dietary counseling were sufficient. The patient complied excellently, and after a short period of time, the objective microbiological examination showed that the actual caries risk had been reduced.

Case 3

E. K., woman, 25 years old. Referred to the faculty clinic from a private practitioner, who wrote:

> The patient has returned again with cavities and need for restorations. At this examination, 37 lesions were recorded. At earlier visits, she had received operative treatment, including endodontics, etc. I have not been able to persuade the patient to cooperate with regard to her oral hygiene. Since I am not able to handle the caries situation of this patient, I would appreciate your help.

From the case history: Mother of two, divorced, works full time as a secretary. Considers herself completely healthy.

Clinical examination: Skin pale and sallow. Several large carious lesions and temporary fillings; heavy plaque.
Dietary history: Deficient intake of several nutrients. High sucrose consumption. Eats throat lozenges.

Laboratory examinations:

Month	Secretion rate, ml/min	Buffer capacity, pH	*S. mutans*/ml saliva	Lactobacilli/ml saliva
1	2.3	3.0	1,100,000	600,000

It should be noted that although the salivary secretion rate was high, the buffer capacity was low. This is an unusual finding.
Treatment: Temporary fillings; fluoride mouth rinses; dietary counseling. The patient failed to keep some of the appointments.

Month	Secretion rate, ml/min	Buffer capacity, pH	*S. mutans*/ml saliva	Lactobacilli/ml saliva
5	2.3	3.0	1,500,000	1,300,000

No improvement. Repeated counseling. In addition, the patient was given treatment with chlorhexidine gel in vinyl applicators.

Month	Secretion rate, ml/min	Buffer capacity, pH	*S. mutans*/ml saliva	Lactobacilli/ml saliva
6	—	—	49,000	43,000

The number of *S. mutans* dropped considerably. The patient stated that she changed her dietary habits considerably; this is the most likely explanation for the reduction of the *Lactobacillus* count.
The restorative treatment was started but the patient again failed to keep appointments on several occasions due to personal problems.

Month	Secretion rate, ml/min	Buffer capacity, pH	*S. mutans*/ ml saliva	Lactobacilli/ ml saliva
14	1.9	2.7	2,800,000	410,000

The values are now roughly the same as when the treatment started. A new attempt was then made to convince the patient that she has to put in some effort herself. The chlorhexidine treatment was repeated before the summer holiday, and the patient came for a checkup at the start of the autumn school semester.

Month	Secretion rate, ml/min	Buffer capacity, pH	*S. mutans*/ ml saliva	Lactobacilli/ ml saliva
17	2.3	5.2	200,000	13,000

The buffer capacity has now increased, the *Lactobacillus* count has dropped considerably, and the number of *S. mutans* is also low. The patient returned for control examinations every sixth month. The laboratory values remained acceptable and the caries situation was now under control.

Conclusion: This case illustrates the difficulties in obtaining compliance in some patients. When the counseling and the practical prevention measures are modified and when the patients realize that their efforts pay off, they become very interested and try to work against the circumstances that lead to the high caries activity.

Case 4

B. A., man, 26 years old, warehouse laborer.

From the case history: Neurotic problems. Takes antidepressants.

Clinical examination: Large cavities in the front teeth; chalky enamel lesions; only the roots of some teeth remain. Large amounts of plaque but no marginal destruction.

Dietary history: Deficient intake of fruits and vegetables. Sugar in coffee and tea. Chews gum.

Laboratory examinations:

Month	Secretion rate, ml/min	Buffer capacity, pH	S. *mutans*/ ml saliva	Lactobacilli/ ml saliva
1	1.7	2.9	1,200,000	560,000

Treatment: Extractions, temporary fillings, general information about the main factors in the development of dental caries. Patient was recommended to reduce the sucrose consumption and not chew gum. Daily mouth rinsing with NaF solution.

Month	Secretion rate, ml/min	Buffer capacity, pH	S. *mutans*/ ml saliva	Lactobacilli/ ml saliva
4	2.6	3.2	1,100,000	130,000

The *Lactobacillus* count has dropped slightly but the number of *S. mutans* is still high.
New information and dietary counseling. Gradually the laboratory values improved. The restorative treatment was initiated but the main emphasis was focused on treatment of the cause of the disease.

Month	Secretion rate, ml/min	Buffer capacity, pH	S. *mutans*/ ml saliva	Lactobacilli/ ml saliva
14	3.1	6.9	1,000	12,000

Conclusion: The salivary secretion rate is high and the buffer capacity is excellent. The numbers of *S. mutans* and lactobacilli are low. The prognosis was considered good and an extensive rehabilitation was done. At the follow-ups—every sixth month and, later, once a year—the salivary and microbiological examinations showed good values. After five years, there were no new carious lesions.

Case 5
K. K., man, 70 years old, retired.
From the case history: Referred to the faculty clinic from a physician who suggested rehabilitation of severely decayed

Principles of Treatment: Case Studies

teeth. The patient had impaired vision and heart and liver problems.
Clinical examination: Cavities in all remaining teeth.
Dietary history: Deficient intake of several nutrients.

Laboratory examinations:

Month	Secretion rate, ml/min	Buffer capacity, pH	*S. mutans*/ml saliva	Lactobacilli/ml saliva
1	0.8	4.1	2,100,000	800,000

After extractions and temporary fillings, new laboratory examinations showed the following values:

Month	Secretion rate, ml/min	Buffer capacity, pH	*S. mutans*/ml saliva	Lactobacilli/ml saliva
2	0.9	4.2	1,600,000	120,000

The *Lactobacillus* count has dropped but otherwise there are no changes.
Treatment: Topical application of an 8% SnF_2 solution in the dental chair. The patient was recommended to rinse with a 0.2% SnF_2 solution at home for two weeks.

Month	Secretion rate, ml/min	Buffer capacity, pH	*S. mutans*/ml saliva	Lactobacilli/ml saliva
4	—	—	1,000	17,000

Prosthetic rehabilitation was performed (see Fig. 11a in color atlas). The caries risk was considered difficult to assess although the laboratory data were good because of improvement of the poor general condition of the patient. He therefore was recalled after three months.

Month	Secretion rate, ml/min	Buffer capacity, pH	*S. mutans*/ml saliva	Lactobacilli/ml saliva
7	—	—	3,600	20,000

The microbiological examination showed satisfactory values.

Principles of Treatment: Case Studies

However, the patient was still treated with SnF$_2$ solution while visiting the clinic and was recommended to use NaF mouth rinse at home. The patient was recalled after three months.

Month	Secretion rate, ml/min	Buffer capacity, pH	*S. mutans*/ ml saliva	Lactobacilli/ ml saliva
10	—	—	1,000	660,000

Conclusion: The *Lactobacillus* count increased and the patient showed up with lots of plaque (see Fig. 11b in color atlas). He mainly ate sandwiches and said that he could not change his dietary habits. He said he could not see the plaque, and he did not keep his teeth clean. The patient therefore was recalled every second month for professional tooth cleaning and topical fluoride applications (see Fig. 11c in color atlas). In this way, the caries situation was kept under control for several years—until the patient died.

Case 6
L. E., woman, 28 years old.
From the case history: Referred to the faculty clinic because of symptoms from the temporomandibular joint on the right side. The patient received regular yearly dental care. She has fillings on the right side of the mouth, and calculus was removed on the left side. Toothbrushing was her only oral hygiene procedure; the patient was not aware of any difference between the two halves of the mouth when practicing oral hygiene. The patient mainly chewed on the right side.
Clinical examination: Decayed and filled teeth on the right side; the left side is completely caries free. On the right side, supragingival plaque; on the left, subgingival calculus and deepened gingival pockets (see Figs. 12a to d in color atlas).
Microbiological examination: On the right side, *S. mutans* constituted a considerably higher proportion, both of the total number of streptococci and of all cultivable microorganisms in the plaque.
The results are summarized in Table 9.

Table 9 Clinical and microbiological findings

	Right side	Left side
Temporomandibular joint	Pain	—
DMFS	37	0
Subgingival calculus	—	+
Pocket depth (mm)	< 4	> 4
Plaque material: *S. mutans* (% of total)		
Streptococci	6–20	< 1
Cultivable microorganisms	3.9	0.002

Conclusion: A case like this with dental caries on one side of the dentition and periodontal disease on the other is exceptional. It happens often, however, that a carious lesion is found on one approximal surface, but not on the opposite in the same interproximal area.

The uncommon caries picture in case 6 seems to be the consequence of quite different colonization of *S. mutans* on the right and the left side of the mouth. In the same way, differences in the caries picture on opposite approximal surfaces can be explained. The reason for the different colonization of *S. mutans* in this patient has not yet been explained.

Case 6 illustrates that the quality and not the quantity of plaque is of decisive importance as to whether dental caries will develop or not. This patient has regularly visited the dentist, and had the cavities filled and calculus removed. The symptomatic treatment, however, has not been enough to reduce the presence of pathogenic microorganisms to the extent that both dental caries and periodontal disease have disappeared. Repeated recurrences of the diseases have not been prevented by the conventional treatment.

Chapter 12

Identifying Risk Groups

Only 10% to 15% of the children worldwide within the school dental service present a high caries activity. These children, however, take up a large proportion of the resources available for dental care. Therefore, it is important to identify these children *before* they develop a large number of carious lesions and, by adequate preventive measures, to stop the destruction of their teeth from dental caries.

In Scandinavia, children are generally selected for special preventive measures on the basis of a clinical evaluation only. It is possible, however, to utilize the salivary and microbiological examinations described in this booklet for selection of children at a high caries risk. Some clinical studies have been performed and the results obtained are of general interest.

In a study in Sweden in the 1960s, the *Lactobacillus* count, used for selection of children at a high caries risk, was selected on the basis of experiences made in connection with the Vipeholm study. In some of the dietary groups, a clear-cut correlation between lactobacilli and caries activity was observed, but in other groups, no such relation was found. The data indicated that the *Lactobacillus* count was fairly characteristic of the individual and that a caries-promoting diet will result in greater incidence of caries in those persons who have an initially high *Lactobacillus* count.

This hypothesis was tested in schoolchildren in Malmö, Sweden. At two schools in the same part of this city all 11- to 12-year-old children were examined for the *Lactobacillus* count. At one school, the children with high counts and their parents were informed about the relationship between a high *Lactobacillus* count and a high caries activity. The children

Table 10 Reduction in *Lactobacillus* counts in children receiving dietary counseling and oral hygiene instruction over a 15-month period

Number of lactobacilli (per ml of saliva)	Number of children at examination						
	1	2	3	4	5	6	7
100,000	0	32	40	43	51	49	53
<100,000–1,000,000	61	35	31	28	21	22	18
>1,000,000	20	14	7	8	8	9	8
Total	81	81	78	79	80	80	79

were instructed to reduce their between-meal eating of sweets and to maintain good oral hygiene. They were then examined every second month for 15 months. When the *Lactobacillus* count dropped as the oral hygiene improved, the children and their parents were informed of this positive result. If the count increased or remained the same, the children and their parents were encouraged to improve the dietary habits. Children at the second school served as controls.

Over a period of 15 months the number of children with a low *Lactobacillus* count gradually increased, as shown in Table 10.

After 18 months, the number of new fillings required was calculated from the records of the school dental service (Table 11).

In the control school, the children with high *Lactobacillus* counts had received more than twice as many fillings as those with low counts. The children with originally high *Lactobacillus* counts in the test school, which were given dietary counseling, received on the average 3.3 fillings each. The corresponding figure among the children in the control school was 8.2. Thus, about five fillings per child were avoided by preventive action.

Because the lactobacilli seem to be mainly involved with the progression of the carious lesion while *S. mutans* seems to be closely associated with the initiation of caries, a new study was started in which the number of *S. mutans* was examined

Table 11 Average number of new fillings per child (after 18 months of trial)

	Initial *Lactobacillus* count per ml of saliva	
	<100,000	>100,000
Control school	3.9	8.2
Test school	4.0	3.3*

*Received dietary counseling and oral hygiene instruction.

in 655 9- to 12-year-old children belonging to the same school dental service outside Göteborg, Sweden. In these children also the *Lactobacillus* counts, the saliva secretion rates, and the buffering capacity of saliva were examined.

On the basis of the number of *S. mutans,* the children were divided into five groups. Three of the groups were considered high-risk groups and included the children with the highest number of *S. mutans* in the saliva. Furthermore, the children in these three groups were similar with regard to the saliva factors studied.

All children including the controls received regular semimonthly fluoride rinses (0.2% NaF) from the school dental service. Children in experimental group 1 also received professional tooth cleaning, and dietary and oral hygiene instruction once a month. Children in experimental group 2 received the same prophylactic program twice a month.

At the clinical caries recording one year later (Table 12) the control children with originally high numbers of *S. mutans* had 2.5 new carious surfaces per person while the children with originally low count had 1.8. This illustrates that the number of *S. mutans* can be used for selection of children with a high caries risk. The children who were given prophylaxis all had significantly less caries than the corresponding untreated control group. The children receiving dental prophylaxis twice a month had an average of 0.4 new carious lesions per person.

The children in the control group who had a large number of *S. mutans* at the start of the study developed more caries

Table 12 Average number of decayed surfaces per child during the experimental year*

Prophylactic program	Initial count of S. mutans	
	Low	High
Control group	1.8	2.5
(no instruction)	(251)†	(51)
Group 1	0.8	0.96
(once a month)	(251)	(51)
Group 2	—	0.34
(twice a month)	—	(51)

*From Klock and Krasse, 1979.
†Number of children in each group.

than those with a low number. The variation in the group was large, however. Thus, the number of *S. mutans* is not an exact instrument that can be used for selection of children with a high caries risk. To determine whether any of the factors, besides the number of *S. mutans,* recorded at the start of the study could give a more reliable prediction for the caries activity a correlation analysis was performed. None of the factors gave a linear correlation. The plaque index in this study was of little value. A combination, however, of a high number of *S. mutans,* lactobacilli, and early enamel carious lesions resulted in an average caries activity that was about three times higher than the mean value for the group. A probable explanation of the phenomenon is as follows:

Large number of carious lesions shows that a person is caries susceptible
Large number *S. mutans* shows that a person has caries-reducing microflora
High *Lactobacillus* count shows that a person has a caries-promoting diet

In other words, this combination illustrates the presence of essential parts within the three main factors: host, microflora, and diet (see Fig. 1).

In practice, the observation should be used in the following way: When a large number of early carious lesions are recorded, a saliva sample should be taken to determine the numbers of *S. mutans* and lactobacilli. If these numbers are high, the patient should be given intensive preventive care. In the study described above, such measures reduced the number of new carious lesions from 8.4 to 0.6 during an observation period of two years.

A third study was undertaken on 14- to 17-year-old adolescents. Based on the fact that *S. mutans* is very sensitive to chlorhexidine, an attempt was made to reduce the caries activity by treating the adolescents with a high number of *S. mutans* ($> 250,000$ per ml saliva). The treatment was performed using a 1% chlorhexidine gel in custom-fitted vinyl applicators at home for two weeks (see page 73). The effect of the treatment was then controlled by a new microbial analysis. The treatment was repeated three times a year, and at each occasion only the teenagers with high numbers of *S. mutans* were treated. Both the test group and the control group followed conventional preventive measures used in the Swedish school dental service, i.e., bimonthly fluoride rinsing in addition to topical application of a fluoride varnish at the yearly checkup when present carious lesions were filled. The test group developed significantly fewer carious lesions than the control group during the three-year study period (4.2 vs. 9.6). A dramatic difference was found among the adolescents who had a very large number of *S. mutans* at the start of the study. In the control group, these teenagers developed about 20 new carious lesions as an average. In the test group, the corresponding figure was less than four. The data from this study clearly show that the level and duration of the *S. mutans* infection are strongly correlated to the incidence of caries in Swedish teenagers.

The findings from these studies show that the microbiological methods described in this book can be used not only for assessment of the caries risk in the individual case but also for selection of children and adolescents at a high risk to caries attack. When the effect of preventive measures is assessed by microbiological methods a considerable reduction of the caries incidence can be achieved.

Chapter 13

General Discussion

The main theme in this book is that salivary and microbiological examinations form valuable adjuncts in the diagnosis, treatment, and prevention of dental caries. It has long been evident that symptomatic treatment alone does not give satisfactory results, and that treatment of the cause of the disease should now be given major attention. For such treatment to be adequate, the factors behind the disease have to be analyzed in a more objective way than has been done before. As an example, some microorganisms are caries inducing, while others are not. Consequently, the level of infection by cariogenic bacteria needs to be determined. Measuring plaque index only is not enough for an assessment of the actual caries risk. Furthermore, the effects of preventive measures have to be monitored.

In Sweden, the Social Board recently presented a guideline for dental health care in adults. The recommendations deal both with prevention, early diagnosis, and treatment of the cause of dental caries and with periodontal disease. In addition, the possibilities of preventing a recurrence of the diseases are stressed. These guidelines are supposed to be observed by all dentists, both private practitioners and dentists employed in the public dental service. In patients with a high caries activity and in patients who seem to run a high risk, an assessment of the causes of the disease is recommended. The Board suggests that in this assessment, salivary and microbiological examinations should be included.

The important point is that the Social Board has taken a definite stand and supported the methods described in this book. The reason is that their applications have led to

General Discussion

positive results in individual patients and in groups of children. At faculty clinics in Sweden, the methods have been used for several years with good clinical results. Samples taken at random show an average of 0.1 new carious lesions per person each year. In other Swedish populations, the corresponding figure for similar age groups is 50 to 100 times higher.

The use of objective methods for assessment of the actual risk has many advantages. Persons at a high risk can be identified before a large number of carious lesions have developed. Consequently, destruction of a whole dentition by caries can be prevented. Where extensive bridgework has been advocated, such work will not be jeopardized by use of preventive control methods ahead of prosthetic care. Furthermore, a patient can be informed about a positive result of dietary changes within a month. Information about the clinical effect — a reduced caries incidence — will take a year.

Also for the dentist, such an approach with positive results is encouraging. He or she learns the effectiveness of different measures and by degrees, and the ability to give the right patient the right advice at the right occasion is improved. Thus, by using objective methods, the dentist can check his or her own skill in the not always so simple but very fascinating art of health education.

In order to prevent the recurrence of periodontal disease, the patient is generally put into an individually applied recall system. How often the patient has to come back to the dental hygienist is based on the results of a clinical examination. This seems to be an acceptable method with regard to a disease with soft-tissue symptoms. Diseases of the hard tissues of the tooth, such as dental caries, are progressing more slowly and lack the possibilities to heal and regenerate — with the exception of the very early stages. The patient with dental caries should also be placed on a recall system. This should be based on the results of objective examinations in each individual case (Table 13). In order to stop the progression of dental caries or to prevent recurrence of the disease, the patient has to reach $+++$, e.g., low numbers of *S. mutans* and lactobacilli and a normal salivary secretion

Table 13 Distribution of preventive measures (according to compliance of the patient)

Compliance*	Preventive measures		Total effect†
	In the dental chair	At home	
Excellent	−	+ + +	+ + +
Good	+	+ +	+ + +
Poor	+ +	+	+ + +
None	+ + +	−	+ + +

*For assessment of the compliance, objective methods should be used.
†For full effect + + + are required.

rate. One patient who has obtained information and dietary counseling might present values from the follow-up examinations that indicate excellent compliance. This patient can take care of the situation at home, and does not have to come back to the clinic at frequent intervals. Another patient, on the other hand, may not show any improvement at all according to the objective examinations. In this case, all preventive measures have to be done in the dental chair, i.e., preventive tooth cleaning and intensive application of SnF_2.

In this connection, it might be of value to discuss the problem of compliance. To comply means to act in accordance with request or conditions. The term is commonly used in the medical literature in order to describe to what extent the patient follows given recommendations. Various studies show that patients to a large extent do not comply, not even if they have a serious disease. The frequency of compliance varies between 20% and 80%. Different factors and conditions influence the result. The physician's most important characteristic is empathy, i.e., the ability to care and to become involved in the problem of the patient. An important way of affecting compliance is tailoring the regimen, i.e., adapt counseling and advice to the style of the patient. Furthermore, it is important to stimulate the patient and to control the effect of the recommendations given. Salivary and microbial examinations are very important in this connection. Without these examinations, dietary counseling, for prevention of dental caries, can be compared to taking a

General Discussion

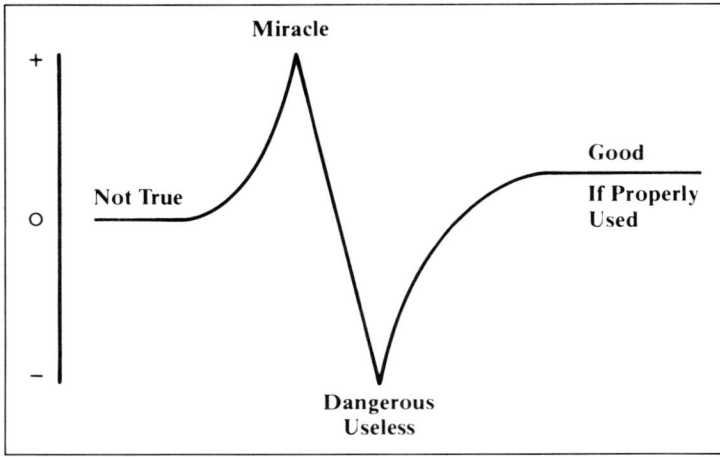

Fig. 8 The characteristic development curve of a new drug or a new method.

course in slimming without using a scale or prescribing an antihypertension drug without checking the blood pressure.

Finally, a word of caution to those who start to use these methods. In the beginning, there are always some problems. New routines have to be developed. Everybody in the dental clinic must know the aim of the procedures. The results do not always fit the clinical picture and the history of the patient. It may be that the methods have introduced a certain error, but in most cases, the results are correct and it is the patient's statements that are wrong. Remember that the frequency of compliance varies between 20% and 80%. Therefore, do not give up; persevere instead! Remember that the development curve of a new drug follows a typical pattern (Fig. 8). It takes some time before it is accepted; then it is considered a miracle. After rebounds generally occur, the drugs or the methods are regarded as useless and even dangerous. Soon a more balanced attitude is achieved. The methods are excellent if used correctly. Try to reach this stage. If you do so, your clinical work will be more interesting and more meaningful both for your patients and for yourself and the profession.

Chapter 14

Summary

The most important information about the caries risk is obtained at the dental chair. The results from salivary and microbiological examinations can, however, be a valuable support for the diagnosis. They give objective information, which supplements other findings, and clarify the approach to treatment.

No single factor on its own implies a high caries risk. Simultaneous occurrence of a series of negative factors, however, increases the probability of high risk.

If the examinations indicate a high actual caries risk, the disease itself has to be treated. The effect of the measures taken should then be checked by the use of objective methods. Thus, for example, the effect of dietary counseling in order to reduce the caries risk should be controlled by microbiological examinations. The effect of antimicrobial measures directed against cariogenic bacteria should also be checked.

Salivary and microbiological examinations can also be used in group studies for selection of persons with a high caries risk. When such persons have been identified, they should be given specific preventive measures. Also in these cases the effect should be carefully monitored by the use of objective tests.

If salivary and microbiological examinations show that the actual caries risk is low, both the patient and the dentist can save time and costs for caries preventive measures that are not indicated. By using objective methods, patients having carious lesions but a low actual caries risk can be identified also. Extensive restorative work should not be planned as immediate treatment of such persons. A large number of

Summary

approximal carious lesions on a 20-year-old, for example, who comes to a new dentist should not immediately have these cavities restored. On the contrary, the actual caries risk should be assessed and further development of the lesions controlled by use of the simple laboratory methods described in this book.

A person with a high caries risk should be recalled regularly and the higher the risk, the shorter the interval should be between one visit and the next.

Further Reading

Introduction

Barmes, D. E. A progress report on adult data analysis in the WHO/USPHS international collaborative study. Int. Dent. J. 28:348, 1978.

Hugosson, A., and Koch, G. Oral health in 1,000 individuals aged 3–70 years in the community of Jönköping, Sweden. Swed. Dent. J. 3:69–87, 1979.

Report on the Working Group on Preventive Services, Canada, 1980.

A Short Review of Pathogenesis

Barmes, D. E. Oral health status of children—an international perspective. J. Can. Dent. Assoc. 45:651, 1979.

Brannstrom, M., et al. Invasion of microorganisms and some structural changes in incipient enamel caries. A scanning electron microscopic investigation. Caries Res. 14:276, 1980.

Edwardsson, S. Bacteriological studies on deep areas of carious dentine. Odontol. Rev. 25 (Suppl. 32), 1974.

Gibbons, R. J., and Quereshi, J. V. Virulence related physiological changes and antigenic variations of *Streptococcus mutans* colonizing gnotobiotic rats. Infect. Immun. 29:1082, 1980.

Gibbons, R. J., and van Houte, J. H. Dental caries. Ann. Rev. Med. 26:121, 1975.

Glass, R. L. Secular changes in caries prevalence in two Massachusetts towns. J. Dent. Res. 61 (Spec. issue): 1352, 1982.

Gustafsson, B., et al. The Vipeholm dental caries study. Acta Odontol. Scand. 11:232, 1954.

*Hamada, S., and Slade, H. Biology, immunology and cariogenity of *Streptococcus mutans*. Microbiol. Rev. 44:331, 1980.

Hugosson, A., et al. Dental health in 1973 and 1978 in individuals aged 3–20 years in the community of Jonkoping, Sweden. Swed. Dent. J. 4:217, 1980.

Infirri, J. S., and Barmes, D. E. Epidemiology of oral diseases—differences in national problems. Int. Dent. J. 29:183, 1979.

Koch, G. C. Evidence for declining caries prevalence in Sweden. J. Dent. Res. 61:1340, 1982.

Krasse, B. Adherence of bacteria to tooth surfaces. Swed. Dent. J. 1:253, 1977.

Krasse, B. Historical survey of animals in caries research. p. 11 *In* J. M. Tanzer (ed.) Animal Models in Cariology. Microbiol. Abstr. (Sp. Suppl.) Washington, D. C.: Information Retrieval Inc., 1981.

Mandel, I. D. Dental caries. Am. Sci. 67:680, 1979.

Mansson, B., et al. Dental health in 13-year-old children in the north of Sweden. Changes during a 10-year period. Swed. Dent. J. 3:193, 1979.

Newbrun, E. The arch criminal of dental caries. Odontol. Rev. 18:373, 1967.

---

*Review article.

Newbrun, E. Cariology. Baltimore: Williams & Wilkins, 1983.
*Sheiham, A. The epidemiology of dental caries and periodontal disease in prevention of major dental disorders. p. 7 *In* Symp., Marabou, Sundbyberg, Sweden, 16 June 1979. 17 (Suppl.) Näringsforskning, 1979.
*van Houte, J. H. Bacterial specificity in the etiology of dental caries. Int. Dent. J. 30:305, 1980.

Case History and Clinical Examination

Brightman, V. J. Rational procedures for diagnosis. p. 2 *In* M. A. Lynch (ed.) Burket's Oral Medicine. Philadelphia: J. B. Lippincott Co., 1977.

Emslie, R. D. Radiographic assessment of approximal caries. J. Dent. Res. 38:1225, 1959.

Gröndahl, H.-G., et al. Dental caries and restorations in teenagers. I. Index and score system for radiographic studies of proximal surfaces. Swed. Dent. J. 1:45, 1977.

Gröndahl, H.-G., et al. Dental caries and restorations in teenagers. II. A longitudinal radiographic study of the caries increment of proximal surfaces among urban teenagers in Sweden. Swed. Dent. J. 1:51, 1977.

Möller, I. J., and Poulsen, S. A standardized system for diagnosing, recording and analyzing dental caries data. Scand. J. Dent. Res. 81:1, 1973.

Dietary Analysis

Burke, B. S. The dietary history as a tool in research. J. Am. Diet. Assoc. 23:1041, 1974.

Department of National Health and Welfare of Canada. Recommended nutrient intakes for Canadians. Ottawa H-58-26/1983 E, 1983.

*Nizel, A. E. Nutrition in Preventive Dentistry: Science and Practice. 2nd ed. Philadelphia: W. B. Saunders Co., 1981.

U. S. Senate Select Committee on Nutrition and Human Needs. Dietary goals for the United States. Washington, D. C.: U. S. Government Printing Office, December, 1977.

Young, C. M. Interviewing and counselling the patient on normal diet and meal planning. *In* A. E. Nizel (ed.) The Science of Nutrition and Its Application in Dentistry. 1st ed. Philadelphia: W. B. Saunders Co., 1966.

Salivary Examination

Ericsson, Y. Clinical investigations on the salivary buffering action. Acta Odontol. Scand. 17:131, 1959.

Frostell, G. A colorimetric screening test for evaluation of the buffer capacity of saliva. Swed. Dent. J. 4:81, 1980.

Kleinberg, J., Ellison, S. A., and Mandel, I. D. Saliva and dental caries. Microbiol. Abstr. (Sp. Suppl.) New York: Information Retrieval Inc., 1979.

Mandel, I. D., and Wotman, S. The salivary secretions in health and disease. Oral Sci. Revs. 8:25, 1976.

Microbiological Examination

Birkhead, D., Edwardsson, S., and Andersson, H. Comparison among a dip-slide test (Dentocult), plate count, and Snyder test for estimating number of lactobacilli in human saliva. J. Dent. Res. 60:1832, 1981.

Emilson, C.-G., Prevalence of *Streptococcus mutans* with different colonial morphologies in human plaque and saliva. Scand. J. Dent. Res. 91:26, 1983.

Emilson, C.-G., and Bratthall, D. Growth of *Streptococcus mutans* on various selective media. J. Clin. Microbiol. 4:95, 1976.

Frostell, G., and Nord, C. E. A comparison between different methods of culturing lactobacilli from human saliva. Swed. Dent. J. 65:553, 1972.

Gold, O. G., Jordan, H. V., and van Houte, J. H. A selective medium for *Streptococcus mutans.* Arch. Oral Biol. 18:1357, 1973.

Jordan, H. V., Krasse, B., and Möller, A. A method of sampling human dental plaque for certain "caries-inducing" streptococci. Arch. Oral Biol. 13:919, 1968.

Köhler, B., and Bratthall, D. Practical method to facilitate estimation of *Streptococcus mutans* levels in saliva. J. Clin. Microbiol. 9:584, 1979.

Larmas, M. A new dip-slide method for the counting of salivary lactobacilli. Proc. Finn. Dent. Soc. 71:31, 1975.

Westergren, G., and Krasse, B. Evaluation of a micromethod for determination of *Streptococcus mutans* and *Lactobacillus* infection. J. Clin. Microbiol. 1:82, 1978.

Managing Dietary Problems

Frostell, G. Substitution of sucrose by Lycasin in candy. The Roslagen study. Acta Odontol. Scand. 32:235, 1974.

Jay, P. The reduction of oral *Lactobacillus* counts by the periodic restriction of carbohydrate. Am. J. Orthod. 33:162, 1947.

Köhler, B., et al. Effect of caries preventive methods on *Streptococcus mutans* and lactobacilli in selected mothers. Scand. J. Dent. Res. 90:102, 1982.

Nizel, A. Nutrition in Preventive Dentistry: Science and Practice. 2nd ed. Philadelphia: W. B. Saunders Co., 1981.

Treating Poor Salivary Values

Clark, R., et al. Removal of carbohydrate debris from the teeth by salivary stimulation. Br. Dent. J. 11:224, 1961.

Nakamoto, R. Y. Use of saliva substitute in postirradiation xerostomia. J. Prosthet. Dent. 42:539, 1979.

Shannon, I. L., Trodahl, J. N., and Starke, E. N. Remineralization of enamel by a saliva substitute designed for use by irradiated patients. Cancer 41:98, 1978.

Reducing Cariogenic Microorganisms

De Paola, P. F., Jordan, H. V., and Soparker, P. M. Inhibition of dental caries in school children by topically applied vancomycin. Arch. Oral Biol. 22:187, 1977.

Emilson, C.-G. Susceptibility of various microorganisms to chlorhexidine. Scand. J. Dent. Res. 85:255, 1977a.

*Emilson, C.-G. Outlook for Hibitane in dental caries. J. Clin. Periodontol. 4:136, 1977b.

Emilson, C.-G. Effect of chlorhexidine gel treatment on *Streptococcus mutans* population in human saliva and dental plaque. Scand. J. Dent. Res. 89:239, 1981.

Emilson, C.-G., and Fornell, J. Effect of toothbrushing with chlorhexidine gel on salivary microflora, oral hygiene and caries. Scand. J. Dent. Res. 84:308, 1976.

Emilson, C.-G., Krasse, B., and Westergren, G. Effect of a fluoride-containing chlorhexidine gel on bacteria in human plaque. Scand. J. Dent. Res. 84:56, 1976.

Klock, B., and Krasse, B. Effect of caries preventive measures in children with high numbers of *S. mutans* and lactobacilli. Scand. J. Dent. Res. 86:221, 1978.

Köhler, B., et al. Effect of caries preventive methods on *Streptococcus mutans* and lactobacilli in selected mothers. Scand. J. Dent. Res. 90:102, 1982.

Krasse, B. Effects of dietaries on oral microbiology. p. 111 *In* R. S. Harris (ed.) Art and Science of Dental Caries Research. New York: Academic Press, 1968.

*Loesche, W. Clinical and microbiological aspects of chemo-therapeutic agents used according to the specific plaque hypothesis. J. Dent. Res. 58:2404, 1979.

Maltz, M., Zickert, I., and Krasse, B. Effect of short-term chlorhexidine treatment of the salivary number of *Streptococcus mutans*. Scand. J. Dent. Res. 89:445, 1981.

Zickert, I., and Emilson, C.-G. Effect of a fluoride-containing varnish of *Streptococcus mutans* in plaque and saliva. Scand. J. Dent. Res. 90:423, 1982.

Zickert, I., Emilson, C.-G., and Krasse, B. Effect of caries preventive measures in children highly infected with the bacterium *Streptococcus mutans*. Arch. Oral Biol. 27:861, 1982.

Fluoride Prevention in Adults

*Keyes, P. H., and Englander, H. R. Fluoride therapy in the treatment of dento-microbial plaque diseases. J. Am. Soc. Prev. Dent. 5:17, 1975.

Koch, G., and Petersson, L. G. Caries preventive effect of a fluoride-containing varnish (Duraphat) after 1 year's study. Community Dent. Oral Epidemiol. 3:262, 1975.

Loesche, W., et al. Effect of topical acidulated phosphate fluoride on percentage of *Streptococcus mutans* and *Streptococcus sanguis* in plaque. Caries Res. 9:139, 1975.

Maltz, M., and Emilson, C.-G. Susceptibility of oral bacteria to various fluoride salts. J. Dent. Res. 61:786, 1982.

Mellberg, J. R., and Ripa, L. W. Fluoride in Preventive Dentistry. Chicago: Quintessence Publishing Co., 1983.

Svanberg, M., and Westergren, G. Effect of SnF_2 administered as mouth rinses or topically applied on *Streptococcus mutans* and lactobacilli in dental plaque and saliva. Scand. J. Dent. Res. 90:123, 1983.

U. S. Department of Health, Education, and Welfare, Food and Drug Administration. Anticaries drug products for over-the-counter human use. Federal Register 45:20666. Washington, D. C.: U. S. Government Printing Office, 1981.

Principles of Treatment: Case Studies

Krasse, B. Can microbiological knowledge be applied in dental practice for the treatment and prevention of dental caries. J. Can. Dent. Assoc. 50:221, 1984.

Krasse, B. Approaches to prevention. p. 867 *In* H. M. Stiles et al. (eds.) Microbial Aspects of Dental Caries. Vol. III. Washington, D. C.: Information Retrieval Inc., 1976.

Nyman, S., Bratthall, D., and Böhlin, E. The Swedish dental health programme for adults. Int. Dent. J. 34:130–134, 1984.

Silver, J. G., and Krasse, B. Treatment of dental caries monitored by microbiological methods. Report of two cases. J. Can. Dent. Assoc. 1985 (in press).

Svanberg, M., and Krasse, B. Asymmetrical dental caries and *Streptococcus mutans* infection. J. Am. Dent. Assoc. 96:1025, 1977.

Indentifying Risk Groups

Birkeland, J. M., Brock, L., and Jorkjend, L. Caries experience as predictor for caries incidence. Community Dent. Oral Epidemiol. 4:66, 1976.

Crossner, C. G. Salivary *Lactobacillus* counts in the prediction of caries activity. Community Dent. Oral Epidemiol. 9:182, 1981.

Klock, B. Prediction and Prevention of Caries. A Study in Schoolchildren. Thesis, University of Göteborg: Akadem. Avhandl., 1980.

Klock, B., and Krasse B. A comparison between different methods for prediction of caries activity. Scand. J. Dent. Res. 87:129, 1979.

Koch, G. Selection and caries prophylaxis of children with high caries activity. Odontol. Rev. 21:71, 1970.

Mandel, I. D. Salivary factors in caries prediction. p. 147 *In* B. Bibby and R. Schern (eds.) Proc. Methods of Caries Prediction (Sp. Suppl.) Microbiol. Abstr., 1978.

Rundegren, J., and Ericson, T. Actual caries development compared with expected caries activity. Community Dent. Oral Epidemiol. 6:97, 1978.

Zickert, I., Emilson C.-G., and Krasse, B. Correlation of level and duration of *Streptococcus mutans* infection with incidence of dental caries. Infect. Immun. 39:982, 1982.

Index

A

Actinomyces 18, 22
Actinomyces viscosus 22
American Dental
   Association 53

C

Canadian Dental
   Association 53
Caries,
   Actinomyces relation 22
   activity 12
   causes of 15
   definition 15
   dentin 15
   development
      factors 18, 19, 26, 51
   diagnosis,
      definition 14
      principles 75, 89, 91-95, 96-98
   diet in 19, 23, 26, 51
   enamel 15
   frequency 11
   host factors 19, 25, 26, 51
   incidence 12
   initial lesion 15
   lactobacilli,
      reduction 63-67
      relation 21, 49, 51
   Lactobacillus count
      and 85, 86, 87
   microorganisms 18, 19, 26, 45-47, 63-67, 91-94
      reduction 63-67
   occlusal surface
      attack 15
   pathogenesis 15-28
   points of attack 15
   prevalence 11, 12, 16
   prevention
      principles 91-94
   risk assessment 13, 26, 43, 49, 51, 75, 85-89, 91-94
   salivary secretion rate
      in 16, 42, 43, 59-62
   starch relation 23
   Streptococcus mutans,
      reduction 63-67
      relation 18, 20, 21, 49, 51
   Streptococcus mutans
      count and 86, 87, 88, 89
   sucrose relation 23, 49, 51
   treatment,
      case studies 75-83
      principles 11, 75-83, 91-94

Index

treatment of causes
of 11
Case history 29-33
  diet 29
  medicines 30
Chlorhexidine 66, 67, 89

D

DMFS 11
DFMT 11
Demineralization 20
Dentin caries 15
Diet,
  analysis 35-40
  caries relation 19, 23, 26
  compliance with 55
  counseling 52, 57
  intake evaluation 36
  intake record 35, 40
  lactobacilli relation 56
  management 53-57
  problems 53-57
  recommendations 53, 55
  Streptococcus mutans relation 56
Drug development 94

E

Enamel caries 15
Examination, clinical, 16, 29-33, 95-96
  completing 27
  intraoral 31
  physical state 31
  radiographic 32

F

Fluorides,
  adult use 69-74
  controls for use 73
  dentifrice 70, 73
  effects 70
  gels 66, 67, 72, 73
  indications for 73
  mechanisms of action 69
  mouth rinse 70, 73
  polishing paste 72
  systemic 71
  tablets 71, 73
  topical 60, 65, 66, 67, 70, 71, 72, 75
  varnish 72, 73

L

Lactobacilli, 18, 21
  determination of 45, 47
  diet relation 56
  reduction 63-67
    antimicrobial 65
    chemical 65
    dietary 64
    mechanical 64
Lactobacillus count 85, 86, 87, 88, 89

M

Microorganisms, acid production 18

Index

O

Occlusal surface caries
   attack   15
Oral hygiene   60, 64

P

Patient at risk,   13, 49, 51, 75, 85-89, 90-94, 95-96
   children   21, 85-89
   identification of   85-91
Patient compliance   93
Periodontal diseases   91, 92

Plaque,
   microbiology   47
   sampling   47
Prevention, aims of   13, 91-94

S

Saliva,
   artificial   61
   buffer capacity,   42, 59
      causes of low   59
      increase measures   59, 60, 61, 62
   examination of   41-43
   microbiology   45-47
   sampling   41, 45
Salivary secretion rate,
   and caries   16, 42, 43, 59-62, 91
   determination of   41
   increase measures   59, 60, 61, 62
   low, causes of   59
Sorbitol   54, 59, 60, 65
Starch, relation to
   caries   23
Streptococcus mutans,   18, 20
   caries risk   18, 20, 21, 49, 51
   cariogenic properties   21
   determination of   45, 47
   diet relation   56
   reduction,   63-67
      antimicrobial   65
      chemical   65
      dietary   64
      mechanical   64
   sucrose relation   24
Streptococcus mutans
   count   86, 87, 88, 89
Sucrose,
   caries relation   23, 49, 51
   Streptococcus mutans relation   24
Sweden Social Board
   Guidelines   91

U

University of Göteborg,
   Department of
   Cariology   60-75

V

Vipeholm Study   23, 85

X

Xerostomia   60, 61
Xylitol   65

Color Atlas

Figs. 9a to d   I.B., woman, 28 years old (Case 1).

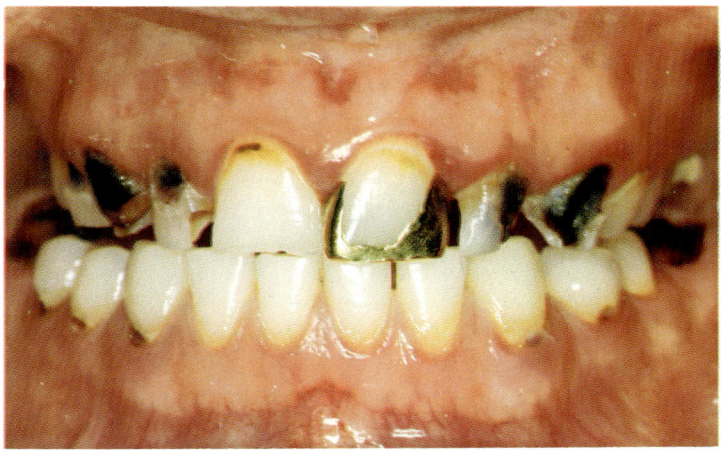

Fig. 9a   The cavities are heavily pigmented and have a hard bottom.

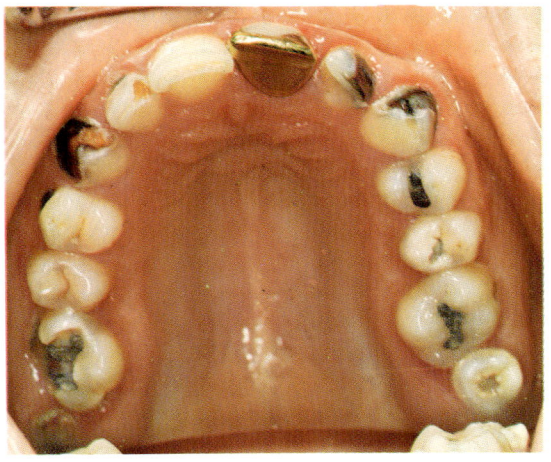

Fig. 9b   Low numbers of *S. mutans* and lactobacilli support the clinical impression that the actual caries risk is low.

Color Atlas

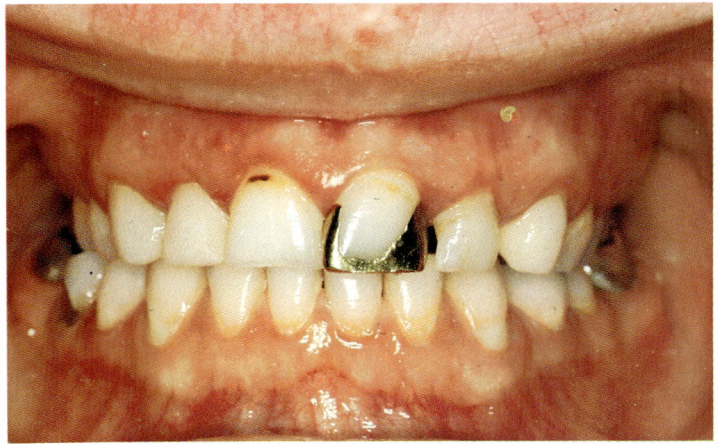

Fig. 9c The cavities are restored. No preventive measures.

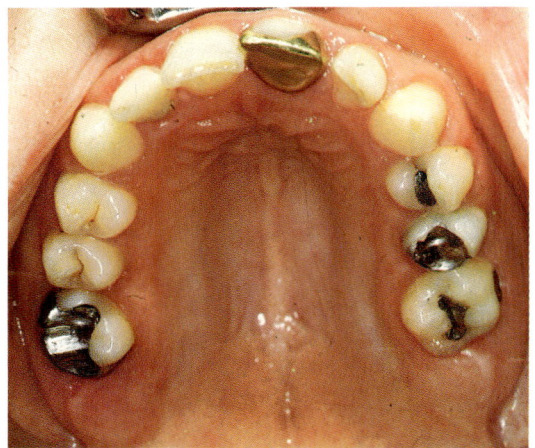

Fig. 9d After two years no new carious lesions.

Color Atlas

Figs. 10a to c   M.L., woman, 30 years old (Case 2).

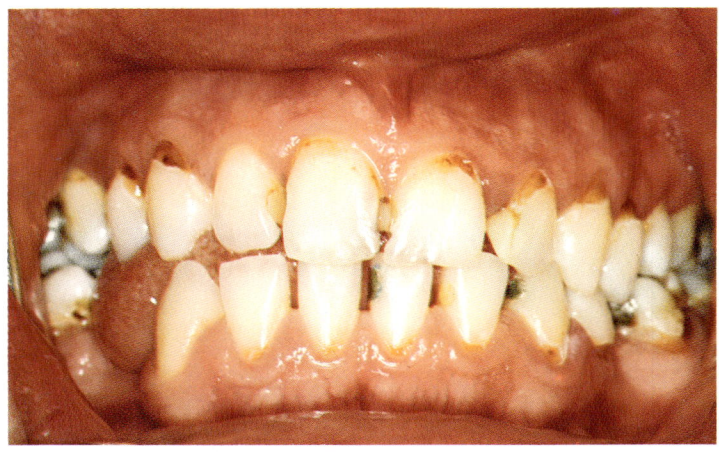

Fig. 10a   Chalky enamel lesions and soft, light brown cavities.

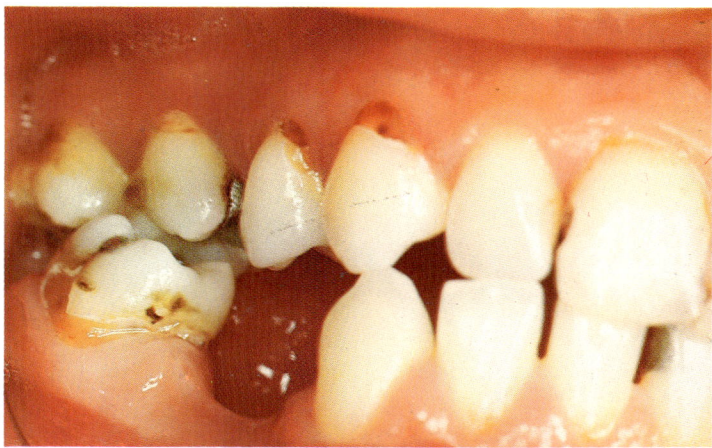

Fig. 10b   High numbers of *S. mutans* and lactobacilli support the clinical impression of a high caries risk. Treatment of the cause of the disease is instituted. The effect of the preventive measures is controlled before permanent restorations are made.

Color Atlas

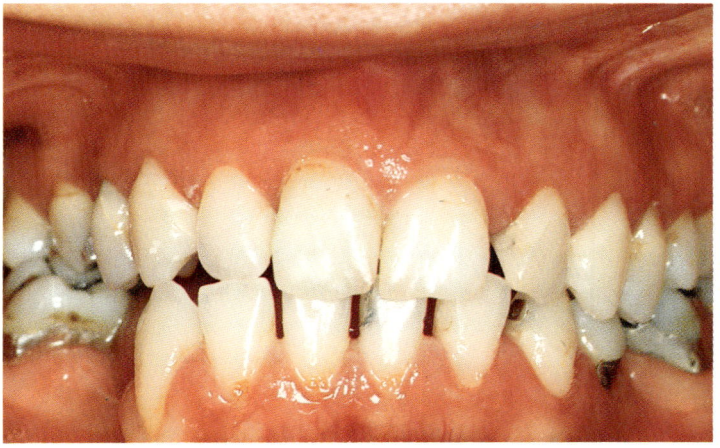

Fig. 10c The patient complied excellently. No progression of incipient lesions.

Figs. 11a to c   K.K., man, 70 years old (Case 5).

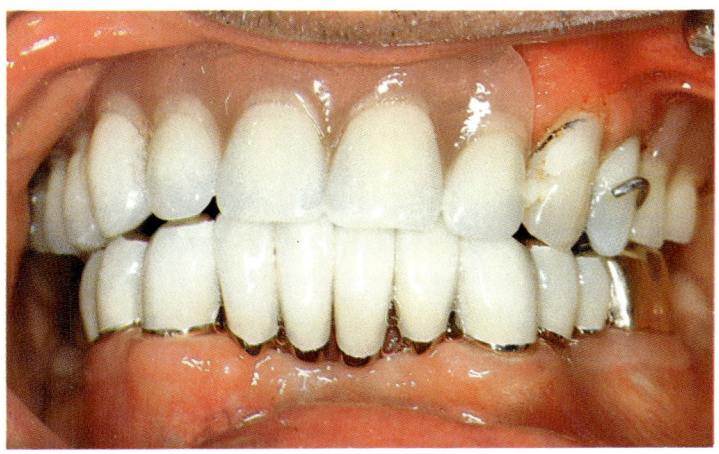

Fig. 11a The caries risk was considered high. Preventive measures were instituted before the prosthetic treatment (full denture in the upper jaw, bridge in the lower).

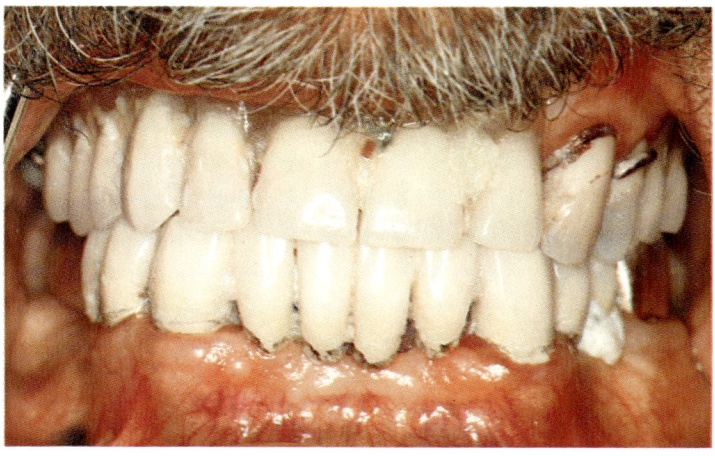

Fig. 11b The patient does not comply. He does not keep his teeth clean nor change his dietary habits.

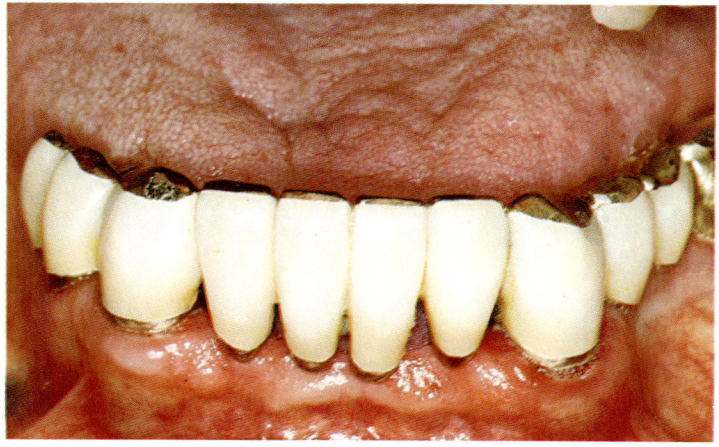

Fig. 11c The caries situation is kept under control by professional tooth cleaning and topical fluoride application every third month.

Color Atlas

Figs. 12a to d   L.E., woman, 28 years old (Case 6).

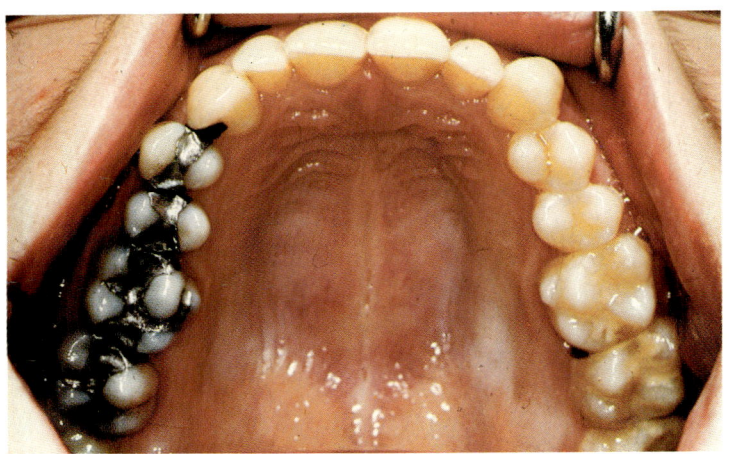

Fig. 12a

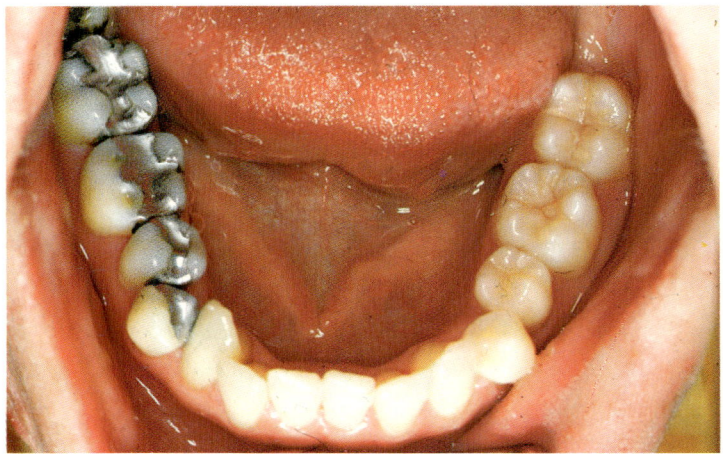

Fig. 12b

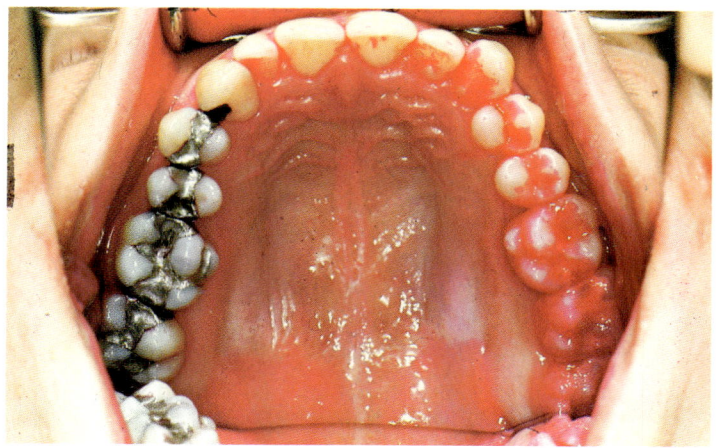

Fig. 12c

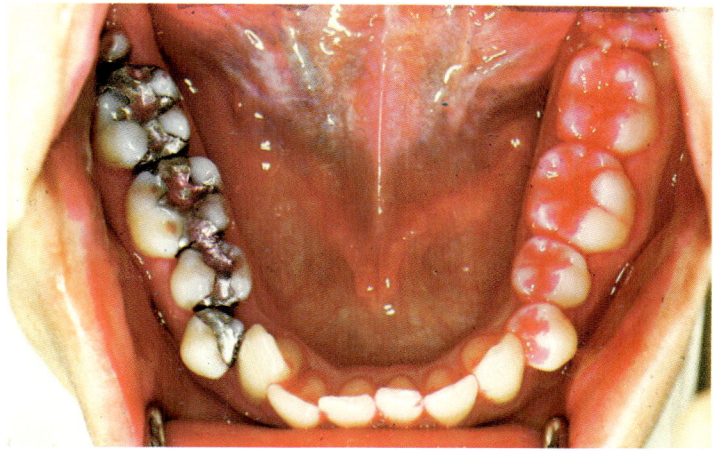

Fig. 12d Decayed and filled teeth on the right side of the mouth. On the left side, periodontal disease. On the right side *S. mutans* constitutes a considerably higher proportion of the microorganisms in the plaque than on the left side.

Quintessential to dentistry.....

Guide to Antibiotic Use in Dental Practice

Edited by Michael G. Newman and Anthony D. Goodman
with 11 contributors

This is the first antibiotic guide devoted exclusively to the needs of dental practitioners. Thirteen experts have pooled their expertise to make the guide an excellent source of information about the use of antibiotics in clinical dentistry. Its handbook format affords quick location of situation-specific information on drug dosages and effects—both adverse and therapeutic.

Selecting the best antibiotic treatment involves matching the pharmacology of a drug with the microbiology of an infection. The book therefore begins with discussions of contemporary infection microbiology, the properties of oral antibiotics and topical agents, modern culture-taking techniques, and the dentist's role in successful susceptibility testing. Systemic factors, another major consideration when choosing an antibiotic, are addressed in chapters on special considerations for women, the medically compromised, and patients with neoplastic disease.

Adverse effect of antibiotics are covered in chapters on antibiotic-induced gastrointestinal problems and allergic reaction. Antibiotic use in the specialty areas of dentistry is surveyed in chapters on endodontics, pedodontics, periodontics, and oral surgery. Prophylactic antibiotic therapy is also carefully evaluated, and medicolegal issues are discussed in terms of the latest understanding of the infectious process.

220 pages. ISBN 0-86715-149-8

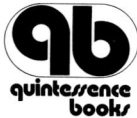

Quintessence Publishing Co. Inc.
8 South Michigan Avenue, Suite 2301
Chicago, Illinois 60603